Cancer Set Me Free

Turning crisis into calm to survive anything

by GLENN STURM

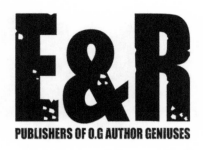

PUBLISHERS OF O.G AUTHOR GENIUSES

Published by E&R Publishers New York, NY USA
An imprint of MillsiCo Publishing, USA
www.EandR.pub

Your guarantee of quality
As publishers, we strive to produce every book to the highest
commercial standards. The printing and binding have been
planned to ensure a sturdy, attractive publication that should
give years of enjoyment. If your copy fails to meet our high
standards, please inform us and we will gladly replace it.

publishing@EandR.pub

ISBN: 9781945674495 (Hardcover)
ISBN: 9781945674686 (Jacketed Hardcover)
ISBN: 9781945674624 (Paperback)
Library of Congress Control Number 2022946155

First edition

DEDICATION

To those like me who wish to leave people,
places, things, and the world better than we found it.

TABLE OF CONTENTS

ACKNOWLEDGMENTS

This entire book is about acknowledgment. Every person who has given me permission to succeed, courage to press on, and inspiration to survive. But let me list a few standouts.

Those Who Have Kept Me Alive

Francine Foss, M.D.

Otis Webb Brawley, M.D.

Sunshine Sousa, RN

Julie Rand Dorney, M.D.

Alexandria "Xandi" Garino, PhD, PA-C

Stacy Hund, PT, DPT, CSCS

Tino (AKA "Radar") Rivera

The nurses, and staff of Infusion 7

Family, Friends, and Mentors

Beth M. McPhee

Jay Sturm

Daniel Sturm

Col. Earl C. Sturm (Dad)

Edith Sturm (Mom)

Sylvia Gort

Jon Mills

Patty Byrd

Randy Talbot

Ken Ford, PhD

Dave Macartney

Rob Varn

Gray Johnson

James Muir

Ray Daniel

Daniel Hodgson

Jerry Currington

Paul Kamstra

Britany Lundsford Kurz

COVER IMAGE

The picture on the cover is called "A New Day." I took it out my back door early in my cancer battle. It reflects that my world has changed. However, it shows it's A New Day and another day to celebrate life, family, friendships, and this wonderful world that our respective god or higher authority god has provided us. I have been so blessed in my life. I count the blessings, but I respect what they have provided to me. Thank you for taking the time to read this book.

FOREWORD

Jon L. Mills, ESQ

**Professor of Law and Dean Emeritus
University of Florida**

**Former
Speaker of the House
State of Florida**

This is a story of human strength.

There is nothing quite like cancer. The word is toxic, and the reality is soul crushing. Glenn Sturm got the call on cancer on January 21, 2009. The message of the call is straightforward: you have cancer.

Millions of us have received that message. Our brains shut down. We hear static.

What Glenn has done since he got "the call" is more than survive. His journey and his message are for anyone who has cancer, anyone who knows someone with cancer and, by the way, anyone who faces tragedy. So, that's everyone.

From the day Glenn learned of his cancer he took a different approach. The goal was not just to survive but to get better at life. This story paints a picture of the world of living with cancer. The diagnosis, the waiting, the treatments, the doctors, the disappointments, the triumphs, the pain, the intensity.

But this story is about much more than cancer. It is about the emotional lessons learned throughout a fascinating life and how those lessons sustain Glenn in the everyday challenge of living with cancer. We can all learn.

We should know ourselves and know our doctors. Specifically understanding our own condition, treatment and effects can save our lives. Glenn's attention to being a smart patient probably saved his life.

But being a patient is not Glenn's profession. A central message of the book is that rather than shrink from life and the joy of living, Glenn made it his job to learn new things and get better. How about running a marathon, becoming a renowned photographer, getting his golf handicap down to two? These are not the actions of sick person seeking refuge and sympathy.

Glenn has been a lawyer, soldier, son, and father. He draws on each of those sources for strength. The strength and wisdom from his father and mother and the lessons of toughness and persistence from the military. Glenn draws strength from family. And cancer forces some introspection. The realities and talk of mortality tend to do that. He says that introspection made him a better father. Instead of shrinking from cancer he embraced the emotions and insights it brought.

A message that we as cancer patients, survivors or humans must take from this book is that we must open our eyes to joy and discovery—now. We are not defined by cancer. Self-pity is debilitating and as Glenn says we must "give up hope for a better yesterday."

The remarkable life experiences and messages that Glenn intersperses with his long cancer journey are more incisive because the lessons are made more vivid by the cancer experience. Persistence in life and in a cancer journey are indispensable. Cancer is persistent. It does not take a day off. Glenn's journey personifies persistence, determination, and courage. His journey includes an understanding of the various parts of the cancer experience that, as it turns out, mirror the trials of life. How painful is the uncertainty of delayed diagnosis? How disturbing is the knowledge that you will get chemotherapy the rest of your life? Well, it depends. No self-pity. Work out every day and schedule joyful things to do. Climb a mountain. Photograph a solar eclipse in Patagonia. That is Glenn's approach.

Glenn shares feeling and regrets. He regrets the day he didn't take a walk around the lake with his grandson. His regret makes us feel and makes us think about our own decisions.

In 2023 Glenn faces squarely his next challenges. He is committed to improving his golf game and playing in the British Amateur. He is committed to a better tomorrow and that is the lesson this book teaches each of us who are survivors of life. Tomorrow is a joyous opportunity. Take it.

PROLOGUE

By Simon Mills, E&R Publishers, New York

Success, power, and happiness are all independent of each other. They are well and good while you have your health. When your doctor tells you that you have a significant medical condition and your health declines, you look back on these elements through a very different lens. This book offers to take you on a vicarious journey through a life of wealth, stealth, abundance, privilege, power, and other curses. To whom much is given, much is required, but sometimes, those who give abundantly of time and resources do not necessarily receive an easy ride from the universal forces. If you can end this book with a new way of looking at your own life—at a time that it can benefit you or others— then you have won.

If this book inspires you to do things you may never have done—because you are sailing along smoothly in ignorant bliss, when out of the sky, you are hit with a threat that gives you an ultimatum; give up or meet it head-on—then the author will have achieved his goal.

The author is an unusual spirit. A unique being with a driving thirst to help others. If forces conspired to award him with rare and incurable cancer, then one wonders if that too was a strategic move to open more ears and hearts to his story so that they may also benefit from his influence, mind, and intention. You will hear stories of presidents, promotion, premonition, and prognosis. You will meet influential CEOs and lawyers with stories you'll hardly believe. You will explore the wonders of life through a lens both figuratively and literally as you discover decades of some remarkable photographic art. But it all begins in Iowa City, Iowa, where the author was born and lived for a very exciting three weeks before taking off on an adventure that would significantly affected lives. The author hopes you will join those ranks as he shares an unexpected, inimitable, and—he may say—undeserved life of blessing, no matter its precipitous challenges. We begin.

INTRODUCTION

Well, I certainly am excited to be here. I truly mean that because many thought I was destined for gone-ness, including myself. More than once people who I have run into and hadn't seen in a while were shocked that I was still alive. It always makes me think of that wonderful quote attributed to Mark Twain: "The reports of my death have been greatly exaggerated."

I am now in my 14th year on chemo. I've had 45 suregries, over 500 IV sessions, and over 5,000 days taking chemo pills. That's just crazy. The only thing I know for sure is that I am blessed. I have been blessed my entire life. I was born in the United States and not in a country like Somalia. I had wonderful grandparents, parents, family, friends, and mentors. I was blessed with a good brain, some artistic talent, and more opportunities than anyone has a right to. I'm blessed to be alive, and I intend to set a record for the most days on chemo in history while Celebrating Life every day.

As you read in the prologue—which was written by someone other than me because I would never have said those things about myself—I was born in Iowa City in 1953. My dad was a professor of military science at the University, but it seems that as soon as I was born, the Army decided it was time to move, and three weeks later, we were on the road to Fort Benning, Georgia followed closely by Berlin, Germany and many other places. In all, I went to 12 schools from K-12 including 4 high schools.

Moving as much as we did, gave me the advantage of being able to approach people I'd never met more and more easily. It was just a function of survival, and I got good at it which has served me my whole life.

Relationships are a powerful force and being able to form them quickly, create the right impression, and make an impact are skills that would greatly serve anyone hoping to do anything. However, these relationships were routinely disrupted. That made them wonderful but shallow.

After a time, I was numb to the disruption and came to expect it. Perhaps even look forward to it. Some places we landed I certainly looked forward to leaving right away I can tell you but let's keep it on the positive.

One of the additional benefits of the regular transplant is the opportunity to be other people. When you are young, once people meet you, you are locked into a particular mold and they don't give you permission to be anyone else, but with new friends to meet every year or two, you can try on different clothes both in fashion and personality. I used this as a wonderful tool to really discover who I was. I was the first person to wear jeans in high school in Ohio and I was voted best dressed in Florida. That would have surprised my Ohio buddies.

One summer, my dad and mom decided to take a tour of Europe, and we were going to drive with my two sisters and a German Shepherd in the back seat and mom and dad in the front seat of a Volkswagen Beatle. I was between four and five, and my mom knew that something had been done to keep me occupied, or I would end up pulling my sister's hair, misbehaving, and generally driving everybody in the car nuts. So, Mom bought me a Brownie camera and spent a couple of weeks teaching me how to shoot with it—that one event and gesture started me on a life-long journey with photography that has played a very important role in this phase of my journey.

I have played golf my entire life. I also played basketball, and football, albeit I was not good at either. Please remember that Sturms never quit. I also earned my Eagle Scout. The title Eagle Scout, much like Governor or President, is held for life hence the term "Once an Eagle, always an Eagle," and I suppose those principles still guide me as they did back then. Golf, too, stayed with me, and to this day, I play a reasonably high level of the game. It doesn't hurt that I now live on one of the most beautiful golf courses in the world. I love to golf so much that it has led me to some wonderful experiences, such as having the honor to play and spend some time with the likes of Arnold Palmer and Lee Trevino. I was also honored to spend some time with Nick Price; a true gentleman. I learned so much from my time with them and I am still learning from them.

I was lucky picking my college. Just before my senior year in high school, we moved to Florida. At the start of the school year I was informed that I had to take an achievement test. I treated the Florida Placement Test as a joke, but I got a perfect score. I picked the University of Florida and I applied for summer admission because I wanted to get out of the house and not be told what to do. That was a very lucky and fortunate decision. I met people at UF without whom I would not have had the success in life that I did in college. Total education is BSBA UF undergrad, 18 months at Pepperdine for my master's degree, and then back to UF for my law degree.

As an Army brat, I didn't want anything to do with the Army, but with a draft lottery number of 33, I had little chance of avoiding it. My choice was between being drafted and accepting an ROTC scholarship. The Army paid for my college and master's, and the GI Bill paid for my law degree. Where I ended up among the very top of my class, but it was not without its challenges.

After my first semester of law school, I had a lot of interviews. I had done well in the Army and in business, so people wanted to talk to me. However, when interviewing for internships, I found that people weren't calling me for follow-up interviews. I was very lucky. A friend who had gone straight to law school told me the reason. I wasn't in the top 10% of my class at the end of my first semester, I was only in the top third of the class. I thought the top third was pretty good but apparently not good enough.

That process taught me a wonderful lesson, and I learned it early enough to change habits and end up among the very top of my class. I did well enough that a few decades later, the University brought me back to teach Corporate Finance and Decision Making at the Law School.

Learning critical thinking is the foundation of law. Being a good lawyer is about solving problems, and I have somehow always possessed an inherent problem-solving ability. I am a blessed man.

All of these wonderful lessons and education prepared me to be successful in business and life, but they didn't prepare me for the shock of being told on the phone that I had an incurable cancer.

THE CALL

It was 2:05 PM Wednesday, January 21, 2009. I was sitting at the Atlanta airport waiting for a flight to Raleigh, NC. I was on my way to another meet and greet. Another day, another business development meeting. While I enjoy meeting new people and learning about their businesses, the only reason that I was attending this one was to support a partner who was returning to the firm. While he was a long-standing business colleague whom I was happy to support, I didn't expect anything to come from this trip, and I was a little resentful about having to go. As it turns out, I was wrong. It was a great meeting and a wonderful group of people. But I had no idea what the day had in store for me.

I normally send unidentified calls to voice mail. For some reason- perhaps because I was distracted while navigating the airport-I took this one. It was the call that nobody wants or ever expects to receive. It was Dr. Galloway. Her message was simple, "The biopsy was positive for lymphoma." My response was simple:

"What?"

"The biopsy was positive for lymphoma." She repeated herself.

"Can you come back in tomorrow for additional biopsies?"
"Sure, what time? By the way, what did you just say?"

You can never imagine how you will react to "The Call." My reaction was denial, followed by confusion. I must have asked three times for her to repeat herself. I then figured out what was going on. Since I have several friends who are MDs, I surmised it was a practical joke. My friends are not beyond pulling my leg, so the fourth time, I asked her, "What did you say, and who put you up to this joke?" She quietly and seriously assured me that it was no joke.

What happened next was a roller coaster of emotions. Fear set in; what does this mean? Am I dying? I was a total mess. Who do I call? What do I say? What did I do to deserve this? This total roller coaster of emotions happened in about 45 seconds, and it continues to this day. It surely was the call I will never forget.

The next thing I did was to call my wife, who is one of the smartest individuals I have ever met and generally a very practical person. Unless, of course, she is looking at shoes, in which case she has never met a pair of Manolo Blahniks that she didn't think was a good deal. When I told her, she was initially in shock like me; however, unlike me, she immediately went to work. Unlike me, she had a problem to solve. I was in shock, not functioning, and she was in her element. Two hours later, I landed in Raleigh. She had researched the disease, knew the science, and had a plan on how to deal with the problem.

The only issue was that I hadn't identified the real problem. The disease wasn't the problem. As it turns out, I was the problem. My whole life has been about solving other people's problems, not mine. I had defined myself by my job and by building businesses. My life's focus was building a career, a reputation, and becoming successful. It was about taking care of clients' issues and sometimes my kids' issues. I ignored my issues by burying myself in other people's problems, and as a result, I wasn't taking care of my family or myself. I was a stress junkie.

This was a wonderful, enlightening, and confusing conclusion to reach. I was starting a journey where I didn't know where I was, and I couldn't see a destination.

The first week was denial. I wasn't ready to deal with the issue. Thursday, I flew to Wyoming to see the family and didn't talk about the issue. Heck, I just didn't talk. I was very tightly bound up and could not express myself. It was painful for everyone around me. I wasn't worth being around.

That weekend I started researching on the Internet. The most amazing thing that I found was an article from an individual who died from the disease. He was grateful for the time. He relayed in his article that, unlike his friends who died suddenly in automobile accidents, from heart attacks, or during the war, he had time, and he was grateful for that time. He stated that, while he was dying, he had time to tell his family that he loved them, and he had time to put his issues to rest. While he'd completed his journey some time ago, he taught me that I was just starting my journey, a journey to heal my mind, my body, and my relationships.

Emotions are interesting. For me, they feed off each other. When I am down, I tend to stay that way. When I break out of the downer, I am at the top of the world and generally stay that way.

At the start of the second week, I decided to make an unscheduled trip to see my wife and Daniel. I was so excited, the previous Saturday I had gone skiing with Daniel. We had raced, and it was one of the best days of my life. At the end of the race, I had to explain to my 8-year-old expert snowboarding son that the reason his father, a 55-year- old novice skier, had beaten him was that I weighed 100 pounds more than him. He promised to beat me the next time we hit the mountain. That day was a true high.

The following week was great, and I was going back for seconds. The uncertainty about the disease didn't seem to faze me. I was on a high and looking forward to seeing Daniel and my wife. I flew to Jackson, got off the plane, and was looking forward to hugging my wife and Daniel and seeing our dogs Banjo and Gavin. I was excited.

As I was walking on clouds, which turned out to be just the tarmac, I hit black ice, slid, twisted my knee, and heard a loud pop. I had just torn my ACL. As I was lying on the ground, I said to myself, "What more do I have to take?" I had just gone from the most amazing high into a black hole. I had just finished rehabbing from knee surgery, and while I was laying on the ice, I started feeling sorry for myself. It took a few minutes of laying on the ice to develop an understanding of what my daughter had taught me: the "wahmbulance" was gone. It was time to pick myself up, dust myself off, and get going.

I was now at the start of the third week of the process. A light bulb had gone on. While it took a few hours after getting myself up off the ice to develop an initial understanding of my new environment and myself, I believed that I now had that understanding. Heck, my wife when talking to her friends about the issues that I had been facing, joked to her friends by saying, "Maybe it's time to take him to the Spring Creek Animal Clinic and have him put down." Supportive, right?

You can never imagine how you will react to "The Call." I now knew that I was starting a journey, and the destination was mine to decide. While I didn't know how I would conduct myself each day as I faced this journey, I knew that I was creating my destination, and it was going to be great for as long as I had!

Taking Charge & Responsibility
Access to the Specialist

After The Call of January 21, 2009, I had to have follow-up biopsies to confirm the diagnosis. Those biopsies happened on January 22nd or the 23rd. This time the results came back very quickly. They were positive; I had non-Hodgkin's lymphoma. In fact, it was the incurable type. The doctor also told me that I needed to have a specialist in my type of cancer because she didn't treat this particular variety. She also stated that her office was trying to schedule an appointment with the local specialist.

One of the hardest things about medical care is waiting. Waiting for test results, waiting to get appointments scheduled, and waiting to have questions answered are the most difficult parts of being a patient. I can't overstate how psychologically difficult it is for a person to get the results of a test that may show a life-threatening condition and then must wait and wait.

When I hadn't heard from my first doctor's office about scheduling an appointment after a few weeks, I called the office. I was told that they still hadn't been able to obtain an appointment for me, but they were still working on it. As I mentioned earlier, one of the hardest things about medical care is waiting for everything. In this case, I had been told I had incurable cancer and couldn't get an appointment with a doctor. I had to do something different.

I had a good acquaintance, Otis Brawley MD, who held a position where he had significant influence over cancer policy and research. Historically, we would schedule calls, and I had never made an unscheduled call. This time I did. I made an impromptu call, and even though he was in a major meeting, he answered by saying, "Glenn, what's wrong?" I quickly told him, and he said that after this meeting was over, he would identify the best doctor in the world for my condition.

He called back in an hour. He told me that he thought that the best doctor in the world for my condition was Dr. Francine Foss. He said that he had already called her, and she had agreed to see me the following week. She said that she would see me any day at any time I could get to Yale's Medical School. He then gave me her cell phone number. Just getting the appointment reduced my stress. The following week I went to see her, and she is still my doctor today.

What I learned from that interaction was that I had a tremendous responsibility for the results of my care. I had to become involved. It was my responsibility to find out everything about my disease and my current conditions that I could. I had to make sure that I had the best doctors and that I was complying with the protocols that the doctors had prescribed. I believe that one of the reasons I am alive today is my active participation in my treatments.

This belief was confirmed at two different times during almost 14 years. One of the two most significant adverse health developments happened in 2013. Early that year, I was dealing with some significant pain and neuropathy. I had been treating these problems by taking Aleve. My neuro-oncologist didn't like me taking Aleve, so he prescribed Tramadol. He saw me again in three weeks and doubled the dosage of the Tramadol. Everything seemed OK. About six weeks later, I started having liver failure. My AST and ALT levels started rising, and the rate of change was increasing dramatically. I was assigned a liver doctor, and we started conducting test after test. They included biopsies. The hospital consulted with other world-renowned experts. They couldn't identify what was causing the liver problems, and the result was that I was put on the liver transplant list.

I didn't understand the issue, so I started investigating it myself. I looked for any changes in life habits, medical changes,

and anything that may have changed. The first thing that I iden-
tified was the change in my med cocktail from Alive to Trama-
dol. I created a timeline and chart of all my blood tests and then
layered the change in medications. What I found was that after a
delay of a few weeks, there was an increase in my AST and ALT
levels. It appeared that there was a correlation between the med-
ication change and the onset of the liver issue.

On my next trip back to Yale, I met with the doctors, showed
them the data and told them about the correlation. They imme-
diately dismissed my conclusions. They said the "literature"
didn't show any possibility that the medication change could
be the cause. They said that it's not unusual to have correla-
tions without causation. I then asked them what was causing
the liver problem. They said they didn't know and that they
were still researching. At the end of that conversation, I said:
"after four years with no change in medications, we changed to
Tramadol. Tramadol was the only change that I could identify
in my life, including all medical treatment changes, and they
appeared to me to be related. Therefore, I am going to stop
taking Tramadol and see what happens." The doctors said OK,
they couldn't see how that could hurt.

What happened? On my next visit to Yale, my AST and ALT
levels had stabilized. While they were still very high, the increases
had stopped. That was just ok news because the levels were still
way too high. Three weeks later, my AST and ALT levels had
gone down dramatically and were almost normal. Three weeks
after that, they were completely normal.

The second affirmation of my personal research occurred
from 2018 to 2022. It took longer to identify the cause of my
seven eye surgeries. It took thousands of my hours to identify
the correlation, but once again, I was an active participant in
identifying the problem.

These episodes proved something that I knew when this started:

- I am responsible for my own health.
- It is my responsibility to find out everything about my disease.
- I must monitor my current conditions.
- My active participation in my treatment will have a tremendous, positive impact on how well I do with my disease.

SURVIVAL JOURNAL—THE JOURNEY BEGINS

Once diagnosed, I was introduced to an online portal where people in the same predicament could tell their stories and support each other. "The Call" was my first entry in the journal. Chapter for chapter, I will share some history and life lessons, then a chapter from my journal to engage you in the blow-by-blow of my transition into a life of surviving cancer.

Tuesday, May 5, 2009

I have my next Dr's appointment Thursday. I have been having problems being tired. While the doctors were helping me with different prescriptions, I wondered what other cancer patients did when they faced this issue. So, I went to a website and asked the other cancer patients about their experiences. The conversations began with me asking what to do about being tired. The first response went something like this.

"Hi: I've written this many times; I apologize to those who have read it many times. Regarding being tired: of course, you are tired; You Have Cancer! Your body is fighting it all the time, every second, every hour, every day, all the time. Your body is always working to maintain optimal health. You have a type of cancer that is rarely cured, so your body will always be working very hard to fight it. Lie down and take a nap. Give your body the help it deserves."

Suzanne

The following was my response:

"Suzanne, thank you for that very clear message. My wife has also told me that I routinely fail IQ tests. I am new to this, and it is helpful getting honest comments, and I did. I am going to bed. Stay Tuned."

Glenn

Friday, May 8, 2009

I went to see my regular internist today and was once again surprised. That's not always a good thing, but today it was. First, Dr. Kaplan was on time (he always is). Second, he was concerned about how I was doing. Third, he wasn't in a rush. Fourth, and finally, he was prepared. I don't know why, but it seems I have found the kinder, gentler side of the American medical system along with the truly professional side.

I have the same situation at Yale, true professionals. The individuals all care, they are all on time, and I am treated like royalty (are you listening, my wife, Beth, Jay, and Daniel). While I would not recommend it, I believe that it took being diagnosed with cancer to find the best medical care in America. I have also developed an understanding of what quality care means. Most Americans have never experienced it. Thank you, Dr. Kaplan, Dr. Julie Rand Dorney, Dr. Foss, Zandy Garino P.A., Mary Ann, Dr. Owens, Dr. Brawley, and your staff.

Today was uneventful. For some reason, they didn't want to change anything. I guess they thought that eleven prescriptions were enough. While I remain tired most afternoons, they don't think they should change my cocktail for another few weeks. Being a poly-pharma is great; you get cocktails, and the insurance company pays for them.

Furthermore, I thought that when I gave up cocktails in the '70s, I wouldn't go back to them in my 50s, but I guess it's okay if BCBS pays. Blood work on Monday and back to Yale on the 20th. Not much news. Thanks for listening.

STURMS NEVER QUIT

The Standard

People always seem to be telling others what they can't do. That happened in my life, probably just like yours. I had teachers tell my parents that I shouldn't go to college, that I should go to trade school.

In my parents' opinion, college was a given, and I agreed. I had learned as a young man that: "Only you can stop you." More on that later.

My first example of the "Sturms Never Quit" mantra was when I started running ten-kilometer runs (10Ks) as an army officer. It turned out that I loved running. When I left active duty and went into business, I ran these 10Ks with friends in Atlanta every other weekend. I moved to Houston in the early '80s. Everything in Houston is flat, and everything in Atlanta has a hill, so it was much easier and faster to run 10Ks in Houston. I looked at my buddy one day, and said:

"Not this weekend but the next weekend, there's a 20K. Let's go do that."

"But we've never run that far," he said with a little confusion.

"Well, you know what? It can't hurt us. If we have to, we'll just walk, right?"

So we went, and we ran the 20K. Remarkably, it was just so simple. At the time, I weighed around 155lb and was just light on my feet, so I just ran it. It was easy, and we both had a fairly fast time. We finished it, and I looked at him and I said, "there's a marathon in Dallas in two weeks." He started shaking his head and laughing, but I rationalized that a marathon is effectively two 20Ks. We just doubled it to run from 10 to 20. So how bad could it be to go from 20 to 40? So, with no training at all, we went and ran a marathon.

Well, it turns out that the second 20K is a little bit harder than the first. Maybe ten times harder. I ran the marathon in around four hours which is not a great time. The great runners run it in a little over two hours, but I was just dragging. At one point, this gentleman—who looked to me at the time like he was about 80 but was probably 60 or so—came up from behind me. He was wearing a little vest and was running at a slow pace. I guess I looked like a mess, and he must have thought I might fail. As he was passing me, he said, "Sonny, you look like you could use a pick me up." Well, I thought it was such a wiseass comment, but it turns out that he was just being nice, and he handed me a piece of hard rock candy. "Just suck on this and run with me a bit." So, I ran with him for the rest of the race and finished with him. He really lifted my spirit. It was a great time. While there was no question in my mind that I was going to finish, it must have been obvious to him that I had been struggling.

There was never any thought at any time about quitting. I'd be more likely to die than to quit. But that elderly gentleman giving that pick me up at just the right time gave me the burst I needed to finish on a positive note, so it was great.

So, what did we do next as responsible and knowledgeable athletic types? My friend and I got in the car and drove from Dallas back to Houston without stopping.

Now, if you know anything about lactic acid, you'll know that you don't run for four hours, walk a hundred yards to your car, and then sit down for four hours. Imagine trying to get out of the car in Houston. It was virtually impossible to move, but again, you don't quit. So, looking like Quasimodo, on a bad day, I dragged myself into the house.

People who "don't quit" just don't have it in them to do so. If you have that quality, it's amazing what you will accomplish.

In the military, the folks in the special operations community talk about it from time to time. For instance, in SEAL training, the Navy makes it easy to quit. All you do is ring the bell, you're done, and then they'll pat you on the back and say, "good try," and then you're quickly gone. They make it easy to quit, but I believe that the people who finish don't know how to quit.

Not knowing how to quit is one of the things I took with me into business. For example, in banking—some guys get a loan, and you know they're going to pay it back because they're going to find a way no matter what obstacles they hit, and other people will find a way not to pay it back. They're the quitters or worse. It's a very good litmus test to predict behavior. Just look at what people have started and what they've finished, and you'll know if they're hitters or quitters. Just think of applying that little test to everything is amazing what you can come up with.

With the Sturms, our DNA is set up to not quit. Just ask my son. He said to me once, "why did you start this whole not quitting thing? It's hard," and I said, "I didn't start it; it's in our cells." If you really want to know, ask Grandpa.

People talk about the hunter-gatherer diet. Why did that work? They had to kill the meat to get to eat, and if they quit hunting, they would die. That's what I mean when I say it's in our DNA not to quit. Take people in sales positions who are having a hard time making quota or something. You can quickly see the ones who don't know how to quit, who are going to do whatever it takes, legally and ethically, of course, but basically, they'll go to any length to win.

They don't know how to quit. They're going to be successful. It's bankable. Today we tend to teach people that it's ok to quit. It's not!

Going back to law school, I thought I had done pretty well in my first semester. I had three B pluses and two C pluses which, at that time, put me in the top 3rd of the class. Well, at the end of the first semester, I went out for interviews, and I had a lot of them, but I got zero people responding. None, no callbacks. That's when I was told that being top third wasn't going to cut it. There's something called Order of the Coif, which means you're in the top 10% of the class. I was told that if you're in the top 10%, you could be the size and shape of Jabba the Hutt and look like him; you're still going to get job offers because they know you're smart and you work hard.

So, I bore down, and from that point forward, I was at the very top of my class. But either way, I got my Order of the Coif certificate, and I was proud of it. As soon as I had that epiphany, be at the top or fail, there was no turning back, and I had fourteen job offers coming out of law school. I could have gone anywhere I wanted and been hired by anybody. It would have been easy to coast, but once I knew what the standard was and I worked my ass off to achieve it, and I did.

It's not just working hard. It's working smart. It's like that great line by Blaise Pascal, the French philosopher, "If I had more time, I'd have written a shorter letter." I built a plan on how to be successful in law school, and I was. Years later, I ended up teaching at the University of Florida Levin College of Law because of my academic and business performance.

SURVIVAL JOURNAL—MAY 16, 2009

It has now been 11 weeks since my first visit to Yale. I had always hoped that I would go to an Ivy League school on a regular basis because either I was going as a student, or I was taking one of my children to school there. That wasn't going to be the case; well, it may be in the future if Daniel goes to one of the schools.

My first visit to the Yale Cancer Center was wonderful. I met a group of people, from the receptionist to the nurse to the graduate fellow, who were all caring, tender individuals. Dr. Foss is stunning. As busy as she is, she takes time with me. I can't imagine anywhere else where people are that nice. Imagine a hospital where all the patients have cancer, and all the engaging staff has smiles on their faces. And I think I have problems keeping my colleagues motivated; how do they do it?

The first visit was hard to remember because I was in a fog. I had great news; my blood pressure was 120 over 78, unaided. Not bad. Then came the examinations and the workups. Once they had all examined me (three attractive women, by the way), they confirmed that I had cancer. I have FMF, Cutaneous T-Cell Lymphoma. I didn't hear much after that.

My hope had been that the folks in Atlanta had misdiagnosed the condition. No such luck. Dr. Foss talked to my wife and me for almost an hour. She was tender, caring, and compassionate. I remember how she behaved, but I don't remember anything she said.

They provided me prescriptions for Targretin (150mg a day) and Nitrogen Mustard, a topical Chemotherapy. BTW the Targretin prescription is now 300 mg a day. They told me that they would like to see me every four weeks. My new home away from home is a very nice hotel in New Haven, CT, The Study. New Haven is a wonderful place to live, work, play and visit a cancer clinic.

The staff at Yale assured me that the condition was manageable. That should be enough, shouldn't it? However, the next few weeks were very hard. My wife went back to Jackson, and I went back to work knowing I had cancer. I came home each night to an empty house. Where was my family? I had to find a way for my family to be part of my treatment.

Thank goodness for Gator (my golden retriever) and Skype. One of the greatest lines that I have ever heard is, "I hope to become the person my dog thinks I am." I know that I will never achieve that lofty goal, but why not chase goals? The only problem with Gator is his tail. Every time I come home, he wags his tail so hard that it could knock over a chair. Boy, it is good to see him. I have decided that cancer may cause issues in my daily life, but cancer isn't going to define me.

I talk to Daniel almost every day on Skype. We have certain routines; Tuesday and Wednesday are Idol nights, as in watching American Idol on TV. The other nights we try to eat dinner together. I can't fathom life without Skype. I love my wife and Daniel. Seeing them on Skype saves most days.

My colleagues at the office have been wonderful. They give me space, and while they want to ask questions, they don't. It is evident that they cared about me. It means more than you can imagine, and that is so reassuring. That said, at times, I have been very lonely. I have wondered how the condition would impact my ability to work, my ability to think, and my ability to interact with my friends.

I never had to take prescriptions daily. I didn't know how much they would mess with my daily life. The first three prescriptions messed with my routine somewhat but were easily manageable. The next visit to Yale brought a few more prescriptions. I now have nine, or is it eleven? The group of prescriptions is known as a cocktail. I drank cocktails when I was a young army officer; however, I gave them up because I liked them too much. So, approaching retirement age, my doctors decided that I needed to revisit my position on cocktails. So much for being disciplined. One of my many doctor friends now calls me a "polypharma." Well, I guess that's better than being called a lot of other things.

Next week I go back to Yale for my fourth visit. Each visit creates apprehension; how am I doing? Is the cancer worse? Is the cancer better? How are they going to change the cocktail? But like I said, I am not going to let this condition define me.

I have decided to change my routine on my trips to Yale. I am going to use these trips as a growth opportunity. I am going to stop in New York and visit my daughter. I will see my friends who live in and around New York. I am going to go to museums and shows. Most of you don't know this, but I love the theater. I am going to live, albeit with a condition, but I am going to live.

I will report after the next visit. Thanks for listening.

FAITH

We trust people in most cases because we like them, not because they're trustworthy. That's an aggressive statement but take the example of people's trust in their doctors. People have faith in their doctors. I can assure you that you have to have faith if you've got cancer. But the real question is this: is it true faith, a true belief, or is it just convenience? I believe my doctor is the best in the world. She ran NIH's hematology and hematology-oncology, and if you look at her bio, you can figure out that she is one of the best in the world, if not the best. As I mentioned, when I needed help, the chief medical officer of the American Cancer Society told me she was the best in the world for my condition and introduced her to me, so I've got faith in my doctor based on facts.

It reduces stress so much when you have faith in your doc. It changes the whole dynamic because you know that you're going to get the best result that you can get. It's not that you just believe it in a shallow way; you know it! That's the reason I listed this first in the context of faith.

The next thing is finding your true self; what's your priority in life? What do you want to be on your tombstone?

I know what I want on my tombstone, but I've got to earn it because I don't want it to be a plurality or majority; I want the consensus to be that I was a good guy. If that's the legacy I leave—that and a legacy of teaching—then I will have found myself. The faith that I've had in myself will be warranted.

And then it's passion! I don't mean physical passion; I mean mental passion; what gets your creativity firing; what gets you going? There was an interesting study by AT&T. It studied Bell Labs trying to identify why some of their stars were materially more effective in developing revolutionary products or services. The first time they did it, they spent an obscene amount of money. My memory is saying it was around $20 million dollars.

Some labs were creating revolutionary stuff all the time, and others were not. They wanted to find out what was the driving factor for those labs' success and productivity.

They did the study in the '60s, and they didn't find the answer. They repeated the study in the '80s, and that's when they found it. What they found was that the most innovative managers had the "ability to channel one's expertise, creativity, and insight into the work with other professionals." They were absolutely curious about everything, and by being that way, they surrounded themselves with curious people. Now when you're really curious, you're trying to do new things, you create new things. You will fail a lot, but it doesn't impact your curiosity. The labs that weren't doing that were also very effective, but they weren't effective at creating things; they were effective at fixing things. The study went further and studied turnover, and they identified that the labs were not led by curious people and were losing their curious people. They either went to the curious labs or left the company.

Curiosity is an interesting passion. It is a very broad concept. You may be a person who's curious about music, electronics, weather, etc., or just somebody who wants to read for the sake of reading and to learn how good writers work, but you've got to find your passion in order to get there. You've got to have faith that you found it, and you've got to keep your eyes open.

Now, to be more reflective on the subject of faith: we all make mistakes, but we must be able to forgive ourselves and find our need to atone. Atonement is a key part of the path to self-forgiveness. Forgiving others is more about you than it is about other people. It's about you letting go of something. Not forgiving others is only hurting you. It's really hard to move on from being hurt by someone if you don't forgive the person who hurt you.

People don't talk about atonement. I'm somewhat religious. I don't enjoy most of the organizations very much but let's put that aside for a moment. Some of my friends believe that if Hitler had sought forgiveness on his deathbed before he killed himself, he would have been forgiven. They believe that there is no need to atone. I don't believe that at all. I believe that you might not have the ability to atone completely, but you can do things to make it better, and that helps you forgive yourself because you've tried to make things right. I believe that the Catholic approach to the sacrament of confession is a major move in the right direction. The Catholic approach is telling you how many Hail Marys you've got to do. I believe the sacrament of confession is wonderful. I believe that it helps you move past your mistakes and create a better you.

I have a lot of friends who are members of AA. We have lunch each week. One of the folks told me that one of the steps in the process of recovering is finding someone and telling them all your secrets that you are afraid of. One of my friends told me that when he completed that step, it changed his life. He felt free again.

While this is doing something that permits you to forgive yourself, this is not the atonement that I am talking about. What I'm talking about is if you've done something to hurt somebody else, hurt a family member, or have done something that is not right, you've got to do something about it, something tangible. You may not be able to make it perfect, but you've got to do something.

Faith—in this context—is about the wholeness of life. It's about faith in yourself. If you haven't forgiven yourself, you can't have faith in yourself. Knowing you've made the right decisions because you've done the right work. Nobody's perfect at making decisions but getting back to the point about faith in your doctor when you have cancer—this is such a critical factor, and it is a major component of my peace of mind while living with this affliction.

I've got my team at the hospital, where I get several days of chemo each month. The team that works on achieving the best results for me works with me diligently. What does work with me mean? They probably know me better than I know myself, and they really do care. But caring has to be a two-way street. I also care about them immensely. I'll give you a couple of examples.

In my 14th year of chemo, I know most of the nurses that work at the infusion center at my hospital. At this treatment, I had a new nurse; this doesn't happen very often. My new nurse's father had been a battalion commander during the Battle of the Bulge in World War Two. She started talking about her dad and her admiration for him. Pretty quickly, I established that I knew who her dad was. As a commissioned officer for over thirty years myself, I've studied military history a lot over the years.

I thought about it, and I said, "I've got to get you the U.S. Army History of World War II" volume on the Battle of the Bulge." I hunted for the book, and I found an un-circulated volume of it that was printed in 1954. I bought it, and I gave it to her on my next visit. I had my copy of the book with me, and I showed her in my book—which had been used a lot—where her dad was mentioned, and I said, "you'll find other places where he is mentioned too."

The woman was beside herself in joy. She took the book home, and she and her son started reading it. That's what I mean by two-way loyalty. It cost me about $150 for the book, which is a lot of money for a book, but it's also nothing. It helped her become more whole because she'd always heard the stories about her dad, who is deceased, but she had never seen it. I helped her to see it, and it made me feel so good. Something small but carrying this five-pound book around in my backpack all over the place lends gravity to the gesture.

Each year around the holiday season, I come to Yale early. The reason is that I have a lot of pictures to frame. Each year all of the employees at the hotel that I have been staying in for over 13 years, each employee at Infusion 7 (my cancer ward), and several Delta employees get a signed framed picture. Most years, I sign and frame about 120 pictures. You see, I wouldn't be able to fight this fight without the support of a lot of folks. It's a little gesture to say thanks. And the happiest days of each year are when these folks tell me where the pictures hang in their homes. It's not just money but the effort and the intent that carries meaning and builds relationships and, as a result, faith in yourself.

"We Must Give Up Hope for a Better Yesterday."

I don't know where I first heard this phrase. I wish I had created it. I didn't. It explains so much about how we all deal with problems. I can't change my cancer diagnosis. It has affected every aspect of my life. I look back at my first posting when I said:

"I now know that I am starting a journey, and the destination is mine to make. While I don't know how I will conduct myself each day as I face this journey, I know that I am creating my destination, and it's going to be a great journey for however long we get."

As I look back on the fourteen years, I believe that almost every day, I am doing a reasonable job of creating my destination. It's important—maybe critical—that you find ways to aggressively treat the disease while not letting the disease define you. That's an important juggling act.

There are lots of people who will ask you how you are feeling. It seems like every day; someone asks how I'm doing. Today, I believe that it's a different question than the question that we all routinely ask each other. Before the diagnosis, it was just a form of greeting. No one really cared about the answer; it was like saying hi. Maybe the worst thing you could do was to tell someone else about your problems. Today, when I hear the question, it seems different. I believe most people are truly asking how cancer and pharmaceutical cocktails are affecting my life.

Some folks ask me how I am doing it. I don't know what they are thinking when they ask the question. Are they asking how I am still alive? Are they asking how do I go to the gym? I really don't understand the question. It seems like they are asking if I am superhuman. My standard response is that I don't understand the question. What am I supposed to do? I follow my doctors' instructions; I am highly compliant with taking all the meds that I am supposed to take; I work out six days a week and spend as much time as I can doing the things that bring me joy. Isn't that what everyone is supposed to do?

You can't let these questions get you down. The person asking the question doesn't know the effect of being constantly reminded of the issue you are facing. I think it's best if you have a canned answer. My standard answer is that I'm fine. Most of my female friends know that I'm saying that I don't want to talk about it. Most of my guy friends think that everything is ok. Since I've taken the position that I leave cancer in New Haven, I think that's a perfectly "fine" answer. Just remember that cancer will always be part of your history, and we must all give up hope for a better yesterday.

SURVIVAL JOURNAL—MAY 20, 2009

The Fourth Visit

Well, I kept my promise to myself. On the way to Yale, I stopped in New York and visited Beth and a friend Bob Finzi. It was wonderful to see both. We went to my favorite restaurant in the city, Bravo Gianni. Bob had introduced Beth and me to Bravo Gianni years ago. A friend of ours, Gina Bartasi, stopped by for a drink. The dinner and companionship were wonderful. While it wasn't McDonald's, the restaurant will do in a pinch.

I took a metro train to New Haven. It was my first train ride other than an Amtrak train. While it won't be my last ride on the North Metro, I think I would rather take Carey.

Really, it was fine. I had Internet access the whole way and talked to my wife and Daniel.

I arrived at Yale at about 8 am this morning. They were in the process of showing a lot of docs around the hospital, and as a result, they weren't as organized as normal. They did my blood work, and then I went in for the exam. The results were ok. While my lipid levels were great, they hadn't received my flow cytometry or thyroid results by the time I was finished.

As a result of the exam, they increased, again, the prescription level for the Targretin. It's now five pills a day (375mg). They have also ordered another PET scan. I will have the scan sometime next week. I believe that they will continue to increase the Targretin prescription each month until I can no longer tolerate that medicine. Furthermore, I believe that they will also be increasing the Thyroid meds and may provide another prescription for the itching.

Yale is amazing. Dr. Foss and Zandy Garino P.A. are so wonderful. They care. It always amazes me that they take the time that they do when I am with them. As a fellow professional, I know how busy they are. The fact that with their schedule, they take the time to make sure all my questions are answered is unbelievable. Thanks to both of you.

Well, I am on my way to Jackson to see my wife and Daniel. I haven't been banned from planes yet, so it's up we go. Thanks for listening.

Glenn

The Rule of Three—May 22, 2009

They say bad things come in threes, and from January to April 2009, I had three traumatic experiences in my life. First, I lost Dan Hodgson, who, as those of you who have read some of my writings know, was my friend, my mentor, and our son's namesake. The second significant event was my cancer diagnosis. The final issue was when I heard that loud pop in my knee announcing my ACL tear.

I don't know how to describe Dan's loss. He was always there for me. When I was confused about something, he was there; when I thought I knew an answer but wasn't sure, he was there; when I wanted to talk to someone who was smart and didn't have an agenda, he was there. He was my colleague, my mentor, and my friend. Boy, I miss Dan. That said, I have to remember what Dan did and continues to do for my family and me. We got The Hodgson Test, we learned the power of passion, and we learned that anger never accomplishes anything. We got our foundation. For that, we will be forever thankful because he helped define us as a family.

As I wrote in the chapter The Call, I recounted what happened during the first few weeks after the diagnosis. During those first few weeks, I promised my family and myself that having cancer would not define me. To quote my daughter, Beth, the wambu-lance was gone, and it was time to start living. That said, having cancer has impacted me. Wow, has it impacted me?

I am now spending about 8 percent of each month in New Haven, home of the Yale Cancer Center. In New Haven, I have developed a new group of friends. From Robert, my bicycling, drumming, barbequing, and bartending friend that I see each month at The Study, to Zandy, my PA who, while I only see her in the sterile environment of the Yale Cancer Center, I know cares deeply about how I am doing. I have developed a group of friends in New England who have become a wonderful support system.

There's Dave; while he lives in Jackson, Wyoming, he lived in New England before moving there, so I consider him part of my New England support group. As a result of my time playing golf with a New Englander, I believe that I am spending about 1/3 of each month with New Englanders. To this day, my wife refuses to concede that I am a southerner; I wonder if she will now define me as a Damn Yankee?

Then there's my electronic support group. Online, there is a banker who, like me, seems to live alone. We are both afraid of the disease and how it may impact us. She has a wonderful sense of humor and doesn't have unrealistic expectations about what I can accomplish. She routinely makes fun of my musing and me. Sometime in the future, I hope that we will meet her. There's Judy, who has survived for over 20 years with the disease and who gives me hope.

Having cancer has brought me a whole new world of friends who are facing challenges. The challenges may not be cancer, but nevertheless, they are challenges. In the end, we are all the same.

After reading these paragraphs, I am sure that you will understand that I haven't had any real losses this year. While Dan isn't here, I didn't lose him; he will be with us forever. As Thomas Campbell said, "To live in the hearts we leave behind is not to die."

In addition, I have developed a whole new group of friends whom I cherish. To think that I would cherish Yankees. I wonder what my wife thinks about that!

Having cancer is helping me grow. It has provided me with a wake-up call, a call that came while I was still healthy enough to become a better husband, dad, partner, and friend. I have learned more about myself in the past three months than I learned in my first 55 years.

And then there is my ACL which is healing, as am I. Thanks for listening.

ONLY YOU CAN STOP YOU

People are always told what they can't do. You can't do this; you can't do that. My parents were told that I shouldn't go to college, I should go to trade school because I couldn't spell, and I didn't pay enough attention in class. Well, I had no thought that I wasn't going to college. Everybody else was telling me what I couldn't do, not what I could do. The fact that I didn't know how to quit meant I was going to college, and I was going to finish.

The University of Florida is a good university. It's not Harvard, Yale, or Stanford. But it's up there. Currently, it's ranked the fifth best public university in the United States. Not that I am proud about my University.

I decided to go to UF because I'd heard it was the party school. Since everybody had told me I couldn't make it through college, I decided that if I went to a party school, I'd have a better chance of getting through. I believed that I would have the discipline to do the work, and partiers won't. So maybe my work ethic would help me there.

People tell me they can't do certain things, and I simply say yes, you can! You just must make the decision that you're going to accomplish something. You're going to be a better mom, a better dad, and then make it objective, not subjective. Set standards for yourself. Guess what? You'll get there!

You'll always find a reason you can't do something. That's quitting, and that's you stopping yourself. What you do is you figure out how to do it, you decide you're going to do it, and you accomplish it. That's what it's about.

I went to college on an ROTC scholarship. The military also paid for my master's degree, and then the GI Bill paid for law school. My parents didn't have the money, and I had a draft lottery number, so I had to get an ROTC scholarship. Almost anybody who's going to get into a decent four-year university can get an ROTC scholarship, and they pay for virtually everything. When I got my scholarship, I had to serve for four years, but I got through college without any debt. Only you can stop yourself. Nobody else can stop you.

Going back to the navy SEAL analogy, you're the one who rings the bell. Nobody else rings the bell for you. Just decide you're not going to ring; you won't ring the bell, and before long, you will get to the point that you can't ring the bell. Make a decision, move forward, and make it happen.

There's a great Tom Selleck movie called "Mr. Baseball," It has a scene where the coach tells Selleck's character that he's got a hole in his swing, and once the opposing pitchers find it, he won't be Mr. Baseball anymore. He'll be Mr. Strikeout. I am paraphrasing, but I had a hole in my swing too. I couldn't spell worth a darn.

You're the only one who can stop you. If you're passionate about something, you might not be successful initially, but with perseverance, you can find the holes in your swing. The next step is to fix the holes, continue with the passion and accomplish what you want.

When I was in third grade, during a parent-teacher conference, a teacher told my parents in front of me that I couldn't spell. The teacher said:

"Glenn will never amount to anything if he doesn't learn how to spell."

I remember saying, "Ma'am, if that's true, if it's that important, I'll just hire somebody like you to fix it because I'm not going to waste my time."

I said that in third grade. The teacher was not very happy with that statement, but it was so truthful because they don't get paid anything for the great work that they do. That's the way I looked at it. My mother told that story for years after.

It is widely reported that Albert Einstein was initially considered to be intellectually impaired because he couldn't spell. Luckily, he didn't lower his expectations in the way that my teacher suggested. Apparently, General Patton couldn't spell either. Reportedly "Patton would lampoon his inability to spell, once advising his nephew, "any idiot can spell a word the same way time after time.""

There is no correlation between spelling and intelligence. Some people become good at it, and some people just don't care because other things are more important. I do know very smart people who have problems with penmanship, spelling, and other perceived setbacks. The publishing company that will be publishing this book, for example, has teams of PhDs that are great with spelling and grammar, but they can't do several of the things that I can do, including writing this book, because I had to live this life to do that. As Henry Ford said, I don't know everything, but I know a man who does.

SURVIVAL JOURNAL—MAY 30, 2009

First PET Scan

I went to Grady Hospital in Atlanta for my second PET Scan Friday afternoon. The people were, once again, wonderful. I won't get the results for a few days, and those will be a few anxiety-filled days. I will let everyone know the results as soon as I get them.

I've been tired the past few days. That's why this is such a short post. On Thursday, they once again changed the cocktail. It seems like every time they change the cocktail; I have trouble sleeping and get chills and night sweats. Kind of like the nights after watching my first Bo Derek film when I was a teenage boy.

Well, that's all for now. I am going for a slow bike ride; then, if I have the energy, I plan to hit a few balls. Thanks for listening. Go Gators.

Glenn

Sunday Night, May 31, 2009

It's Sunday evening, and I am still waiting for the PET Scan results. As most of you know, I am not long on patience. So, waiting for three days is kind of driving me nuts. The anxiety is heightened because after my first PET Scan; the techs showed me there wasn't much there. This time the techs would not talk to me about the test. "NUTS," to quote General Anthony McAuliffe.

Today my daughter Jay and I are spending an evening together on our Macs. Not a lot of communication, but at least we are in the same room with Gator (my first golden) asleep between us. Jay will be staying at the house for the remainder of the summer. It is absolutely wonderful being with one of my children.

Jay is in town interning with Dr. Tom Myer, who is an ortho-pedic surgeon. Tom is a regular reader of the Journal who has flattered me with comments about my writing. Way to go, Tom. In repayment for his flattery, I am trying to help Tom by provid-ing recurring revenue for him. He has, in two separate surgeries within six months, operated on the left knee once and the right knee twice. It's not his fault; I blame the black ice. But for those of you who like injuring yourselves, he is one of America's great orthopedic surgeons. Tonight, Jay and I got on Skype and had a video conference with Daniel. I don't know what I would do without Skype. Daniel had Fudge in his arms (more on her later) and had just finished a day playing golf. I envy the life of this eight-year-old.

Now time to talk about Fudge. Her first week was wonderful. Believe it or not, she didn't have a single accident. An eight-week-old puppy that doesn't have accidents. We are blessed. Remem-ber when I predicted that she would find and chew up certain "perceived necessities?" I don't know if electrical cords for your

Mac are perceived as necessities, but I do know that the Macs don't work without them. Fudge was two for two during her first week. She ate both my wife's and Daniel's power cords. It was kind of hard to communicate with them on Skype when their computers weren't working. Way to go, girl.

Please check out the photo of Daniel and Fudge with the Miata by scanning the QR code. It was taken before he had to get in the car without Fudge. You know the rest of the story.

Well, that's it for tonight. Let's hope that my patience is rewarded tomorrow morning. Thanks for listening.

Glenn

THREE BIRTHDAYS PER YEAR

As I mentioned, I'm religious, but I'm not a fan of many institutions. Christmas and Easter are probably two of the five most important days of the year for me. When I was younger, it was my mom and dad's birthdays that were so critical to me. Saying thank you to them and celebrating them. Now it's my daughters' and my son's birthdays that are important. My birthday is important to me because it's a day of reflection. I live alone in some ways, and in other ways, I'm probably the least lonely person in the world. I normally don't work on my birthday, and when they were younger, I'd take my kids' birthdays off work; the family birthdays were important to me. It was a day to celebrate their life and to make sure they knew how much I loved them, make sure how much I enjoyed them.

And then the Army's birthday is something I celebrate on June 14, and there's a reason for it. I grew up as an army brat, but initially, I wanted absolutely nothing to do with the Army. There's no way I was going to have anything to do with the Army. When I got my draft lottery number 33, it was an easy decision. I had to join ROTC, I started out in the Air Force ROTC, but I just couldn't do it. I couldn't wear the blue uniform. It just didn't work for me. I had gotten used to the green one all my life with my father. So, I went to the Army.

The Army's birthday is so critical in so many ways. First off, my education was paid for by the Army. It's important to me to respect that. My first mentor was a gentleman who taught me I could do anything I chose to. His name was Colonel Muir. He came in one day to my office—when I was a regimental headquarters company commander—and he said to me, "Glenn, I bought these new computers, and I want you to write a software program that looks at the demographic characteristics of the individual members of the army and predicts their success in their various specialties based on their demographic characteristics." "What? what are you talking about?" He said, "Glenn, it's easy. It's a new software language called Apple Soft Basic on an Apple 2C With 64 kilobytes of RAM. You've got 90 days to have this finished and to brief the senior army general. The first thing I did was to write the title page for the program, which I had to do to begin. I call it the Standard Training Uniform Response Management System, also known as STURMS. The colonel had so much confidence in me that I could do it that I did do it. Ninety days later, there was a software product that was predicting the success of people based on the data input. It was a variable database which means you could add data points to it. It was not a well-written program, but it was a program that worked. I didn't know about documentation. I didn't know there was something called a do loop and spaghetti programs where we have these commands called go-tos when you ran out of lines, but it worked, and he gave me that skill. The Army gave me that skill and that confidence.

Let's examine the Oath of Office for a Commissioned Officer.

I (state your full name), having been appointed an officer in the Army of the United States, as indicated above in the grade of Second Lieutenant, do solemnly swear (or affirm) that I will support and defend the Constitution of the United States against all enemies, foreign and domestic, that I will bear true faith and allegiance to the same; that I take this obligation freely, without any mental reservation or purpose of evasion; and that I will well and faithfully discharge the duties of the office on which I am about to enter, so help me God.

Now, the oath of enlistment for an enlisted person is different. They swear they're going to obey the orders of the officers appointed over them.

"I,_____, do solemnly swear (or affirm) that I will support and defend the Constitution of the United States against all enemies, foreign and domestic; that I will bear true faith and allegiance to the same; and that I will obey the orders of the President of the United States and the orders of the officers appointed over me, according to regulations and the Uniform Code of Military Justice. So help me, God."

There's nothing in the commissioned officer's oath that says you're going to swear to obey the orders of officers above you. The Army is the guarantor of the Constitution. Now, we're not allowed to do things internally, but that oath is so foundational to our country. It's really important.

Colin Kaepernick, who in 2016 knelt for the national anthem, is a good example of what this oath is truly about. I have no use for Colin Kaepernick—the person and what he does—but I will absolutely, positively, to my last breath, defend his right to do what he does. It is so foundational to our country and something we're starting to miss as a country. We owe our allegiance to the Constitution, which says that we have freedom from the government. The government doesn't grant us rights. Most countries' constitutions are freedoms to do something; they give you specific permissions to do things. Our constitution is the inverse; it's freedom from the government. So, unless the government has the right to do something or prevent something, then that right belongs to the individual. Please look at the Ninth and Tenth Amendments to our constitution. They are worth reading:

Ninth Amendment

"The enumeration in the Constitution, of certain rights, shall not be construed to deny or disparage others retained by the people."

Tenth Amendment

"The powers not delegated to the United States by the Constitution, nor prohibited by it to the States, are reserved to the States respectively, or to the people."

SURVIVAL JOURNAL—JUNE 4, 2009

Some Good News

It is, I am thrilled to say, time for some good news. After six days, patience finally wore out. As I am sure all of you know, the wait is harder than the news. I decided to stop waiting, and I went to Grady Hospital today to get a copy of the report. After waiting for a while, talking to the staff, and insisting on getting a copy of the report, I was given one, and the news was all good. The disease has not progressed, and it appears that the cocktail is working.

I'm off to see Daniel, Fudge, Banjo, and Bear tonight. More postings this weekend. Thank you for your concern.

Glenn

THE BALANCING ACT

My Biggest Mistakes

Introduction

When I sat down today, I reflected on this past week. Before the week started, I was really looking forward to the week. Both of my daughters and my grandson were coming for a visit. I couldn't wait to see my grandson. They were scheduled to arrive on Friday and leave the following Friday. I also had a young couple, who were golfing friends, coming to visit starting on Sunday, and they planned to leave the following Saturday. I was going to have the opportunity to play golf with the husband, who is a very talented young professional. I was going to have a house full of five wonderful people and my two golden puppies. I was a bit apprehensive about the crowd.

As I was reflecting, I thought about pictures. As you know, I love photography. On Wednesday night, the couple and I had gone to Grand Teton National Park, chancing an opportunity to see the Northern Lights, which were predicted to be visible. My grandson had gone to bed before we left, so neither my daughter, Beth, nor my grandson, Sam, could go. I then started thinking about my grandson and pictures of him. I wondered if there was a picture of the two of us. I hadn't seen any. Well, there aren't any. The photographer had missed a golden opportunity. I was so focused on all my guests I didn't focus on the one person who was too young to communicate what he wanted. I was disappointed in myself.

I started thinking about how I had balanced my week and the things that I did during the week, but more importantly, the things I didn't do. The more I thought about the week, the more disappointed I became in myself. So, I decided I had to assess the information (the events and nonevents), identify the problem or problems, and then create a solution to those problems. You can't solve a problem until you know what the problem is.

Assessing the Information

In assessing the information, I have identified one major issue and several minor issues. When I look at my personal life, I must acknowledge that I have not achieved my primary objective; I don't have a life partner. It's not for want of trying. I have three wonderful children from two marriages. As a psychiatrist once told me, I am not good at picking women. The psychiatrist went so far as to tell me that I shouldn't get involved in a long-term relationship without the psychiatrist meeting the woman. So, one of the principal questions I must ask is, why am I so bad at this? I also have to ask if there is something that I have done or not done that results in this failure.

In addition to that problem, I am terrible at balancing things. Last week my daughter asked if I wanted to go on a walk with my grandson. I passed so that I could play golf with my other visitor. The number of mistakes that this decision reveals is eye-opening.

One of my favorite memories as a child was going to the water's edge at Bowman Lake in Montana with my grandfather. I remember having my grandfather stand next to me and give me advice while I tried to skip rocks across the lake. I loved those moments .When my daughter returned from the hike, she told me that my grandson had spent almost an hour throwing rocks in the river. She told me that my grandson was as happy as she had seen him. So, I missed this opportunity to build memories for both of us because I played golf with a house guest.

The next mistake was that I didn't brief my daughter on safety matters. In Wyoming, we have a lot of wildlife. They left on their hike and treated it like a walk-in town. While they were on the hike, my daughter and grandson encountered a grizzly bear. While the bear was at a safe distance, it was a scary event. Furthermore, they didn't have bear spray with them, and this could have resulted in a catastrophe that would have been my fault.

To Sam and Beth, I won't let this happen again.

So why did this happen, and why do I continue to overbook? The more I thought about the problem, the more I recognized that I have a real hard time saying no. The result of this issue is that I routinely overschedule. I then started wondering if this problem had caused me other problems in my personal life, like not having a long-term relationship.

One of my favorite statements as a leader is that while I encourage conflicts of ideas, I won't tolerate conflicts of personality. Reflecting on this position, I wondered how it may have impacted my personal life. The simple answer is— yes! When my partners did something that bothered me, I never addressed the issue. I internalized it and failed to discuss the problem. The result was that over time, those issues that probably could have been easily addressed built up. It was like loading a bridge with too much weight. What happens next is the bridge breaks. The principal issue is that in my personal life, I let things build up because I didn't address the problem when it happened. That wasn't being nice to me or the other person involved. I let the issue grow and compound until the bridge failed. It was a major flaw.

THE SOLUTION

The Issues that I must Address to make My Life Better:

The following are the steps that I determined that I must take:

- Politely saying no more often and as a partial effect of this, stop overbooking myself. That can be done politely, but I must do it to start bringing balance to my life.
- Scheduling margin in everything will allow for the unexpected. In my relationships, I must politely communicate when things bother me. I owe it to everyone that I know to politely communicate my concerns.
- Insisting that I listen to other folks' concerns and address them. I know that if I have concerns, then they must have concerns too.
- Finally, remember when a friend brings an issue up, that it is important to them that I must carefully and actively listen to them. True Friends bring up issues because they care

about me. It's not easy to give a friend news they don't want. Furthermore, if it's a big issue, they may be thinking that the issue is so important that they are willing to put the relationship at risk, so they must tell me. If they know about a problem and take the time to tell you, they are a real friend.

When I thought about not having a picture of Sam and me, it caused me to reflect on a lot of things. Every time I think about the picture with Sam that I missed, it will remind me to make good on my solutions plan. I welcome being held accountable for anything in my life and the solutions that I identified. So, if you know me, go right ahead and pull me up should I misstep.

My solution system here is a good example of my problem-solving workflow, so I wanted to demonstrate that. As I have mentioned multiple times, the core of my legal skillset is solving problems, and this is how I go about it.

SURVIVAL JOURNAL—
JUNE 10, 2009–JUNE 19, 2009

The Brick

People continue to ask how I am doing and as I have explained, I have a completely different understanding of that question now.

I apologize in advance for the length of the answer, but it's complicated because the disease affects everyone I know. The short answer is that most days are great. While some are challenging, most are just great days. The impact on my family is more complicated. I have a wonderful wife and family who are so supportive. However, one thing that I have learned is that my family is also a victim of the disease. They, too, must deal with my cancer every day just like I do. They have emotional concerns, and cancer weighs on them just like it weighs on me. My daughters are very frightened, but they are acting nicer to me. See, there is a cancer benefit. That said, I must be as supportive of them as they are of me. So, what's it really like? Well, when I was a very young Army officer, we occasionally had

69

to carry rucksacks or "rucks." This is the Army's term for a backpack. While they were very durable, they were also very uncomfortable. For some reason, mine never seemed to fit properly, it chaffed, and the straps seemed to always dig into my shoulders. They always weighed too much. So, what did I do? Well, I picked up my ruck, put it on my shoulders, and started walking. You kept the ruck on your shoulders until the mission was finished. You just sucked it up.

We all carry a ruck every day of our lives, and on a lot of days, it's not easy to do. How we carry the ruck defines us as a person. Most of us get up, get dressed, and go to work. While we all have burdens to carry, some of us are more able to carry loads than others, but we all carry them. That said, some can carry more weight than others, and some just choose to carry whatever they are given, and then some more.

Before the diagnosis, the doctors' appointments, the cocktails, and the side effects, I got up every morning and, just like you, I put the ruck on my back and started walking. I do the same thing today, except the pack is a little heavier. Someone placed a brick or two in my ruck, that jerk. Some days it seems to be a lot heavier, while other days, I don't seem to notice the additional weight. Amazingly the weight seems to be getting lighter all the time. Why is that? I believe it is simple. The extra weight is making me stronger. Heck, it's making our family stronger. I won't go so far as to tell you that it's a blessing, but I have never felt better about life than I do today. Heck, another brick in the pack will make all of us stronger.

Is it tough? Of course, it is. But negative thoughts won't do us any good. To quote Oddball from Kelly's Heroes: "Why don't you knock it off with them negative waves? Why don't you dig how beautiful it is out here? Why don't you say something righteous and hopeful for a change."

So, on those days that I may not look as good as I do on others, chalk it up to the fact that I, like other 55-year-olds, may have had an extra cocktail the night before.

June 16, 2009

I am on my way to Yale tomorrow morning. Will see Dr. Foss for an extended period on Thursday. I will update you late Thursday or Friday morning.

I spent about 3 hours with an endocrinologist yesterday, and they ran a bunch of tests. No results yet, but the docs did double my thyroid medication dosage. I believe it helped me on my bike ride this morning. At least, that's what David said as he watched me ride the second half of the ride today. I don't know if he let me win or if I just had a good day. Either way, it felt great.

Here is the interim update: the thyroid medicine dosage was wrong, back down to 100mcg, only a 1/3 increase.

Talk to you soon.

June 19, 2009

This will be a quick note. I am at a board meeting and don't think that I will have time for a longer essay until Sunday.

The meetings with the doctors went very well. They couldn't have gone better. For the first time, they didn't increase my Targretin dosage. They are hopeful that they won't have to increase the dosage of that medicine again. They did tell me that they will be increasing the intensity of my Nitrogen Mustard chemo next month, but that's not a big deal.

Thanks for thinking of me.

Glenn

Solutions—Father's Day Weekend

As a young Army officer, I learned that I was never lost. Maybe miss-oriented, but never lost. Furthermore, because of what my father and the Army taught me, I have always believed that if you can identify the destination, getting there wouldn't be a problem. My whole life has been about knowing where I am and devising the path to a well-defined destination. Well, it seems that at 55, I may be lost.

What is cancer, and why has it affected me physically and spiritually the way it has? Several of my friends who have read these journal entries have commented that they believe that my friends are finally seeing my sensitive side. My friends who served in the Army are probably questioning my Hoorah. No, it just seems that I can't solve cancer. The first time that I couldn't clearly identify my destination.

The conundrum that is making me think a lot is the following question: If I could fix my cancer, what would the fix be? Now that's a hard question. I will use future postings to question my destination and attempt to identify how I will fix my disease. Furthermore, I am going to develop ways to improve my environment.

I cherish every day I get to spend with my wife, Beth, Jay, Daniel, Gator, Banjo the Shih Tzu, Bear, our Jackson visiting Golden, and Fudge. I also know that they cherish the time they have with me. Over the past few months, I have learned that the truest statement about children is that old saying: how they spell love is TIME. It's not just quality time; it is also about the quantity of time we spend with each other. One of the most significant commitments that I have made to myself is that I will take time for my family and myself. I believe that one of the major environmental reasons that I will improve is the significant increase in the amount of time I will spend with my family.

I have also learned the value of a good dog. Gator the golden is a wonderful friend. He loves everyone he sees, especially me. A few months ago, I gave him his first real bone. He carried that bone around for a week until it was gone. Boy, he was happy, and I loved his continuous smile.

For the first time, I felt I had done something for Gator, like the things that he does for me. As I have said before, I hope to be the person that my dog thinks I am. I am working on it, but I'm not there yet. By the way, don't you think our family needs a few more dogs? I believe that our dogs will also provide an environmental stimulus for my recovery.

While I have been writing this for a while, I am posting it on the Friday of Father's Day weekend. As a result, I have a few more things to say. To dad, thank you. You have been and forever will be my foundation. As a leader, I say things each day that I heard you say more than 40 years ago. To Beth, Jay, and Daniel, I love each of you. I hope that I will be your foundation as my dad was mine. It doesn't matter what the subject is, please talk to me. Like Gator's love for me, my love for you is unconditional. Just like Gator, every time I see you, I am wagging my tail. My wife is the love of my life. I miss you every day we are apart. I thank each of you for being you and for augmenting the foundation that my parents provided me.

Am I lost? I no longer feel that I am. While I may be miss-oriented, I am working hard to find my destination. It's a lot closer than I thought it was a few months ago. Thanks for listening.

Glenn

TRUST

Trust is one of the most powerful emotions and elements in a relationship. An organization that is based on well-founded trust normally succeeds. Trust that is well founded is extremely liberating, and it can provide a security blanket for a relationship and a business. However, some of the greatest mistakes that I have made in business have come as the result of trusting someone where the person or the organization turns out to be not trustworthy. After making many mistakes by inappropriately trusting individuals—and losing a lot of money as a result—I studied my reasons for trusting these individuals and found out why I was making these mistakes. I was trusting people without any basis for that trust. Since then, I have found that most people trust individuals and businesses without any foundation for that trust. All too often, trust is unearned, and, as a result, it may be misplaced. Please test this theory. Whenever someone says they trust someone, ask why they trust the person or organization. See if there is a basis for that trust.

About a decade ago, I had, for the first time, developed a sum of money that I needed to have professionally managed.

I was working with a senior officer at a private bank and believed that she was both capable and trustworthy. The woman introduced me to the money managers at her bank, and I intuitively trusted these managers. Over several weeks we reviewed the rules that I wanted them to follow in making the investments. There were both written and oral instructions. Needless to say, the money managers didn't follow my instructions, and they lost about 70% of the money they invested. I asked for and received a meeting with the senior officer of the bank who ran the investments area.

At the meeting, he told me that the oral instructions never happened and that it didn't matter anyway because the only thing that mattered was the document, the written instructions. He effectively told me I could just pound sand. At that point, my banker, who had been at the meetings with me, said: Mr. Sturm made those instructions, and we agreed to them. Furthermore, she said she was willing to testify on my behalf if I chose to sue the bank.

Her personal courage was both refreshing and inspiring. As a result of this episode, I learned two things. First, I could trust my personal banker. Second, I couldn't trust the senior executive, the bank, or for that matter, almost any organization. My trust in both my personal banker and the bank had been made without any basis. I was right once but wrong the other time, and as a result, I lost a lot of money. To this day, my personal banker is a trusted friend, and I won't do anything with that bank or the other senior officer. It was a very expensive lesson.

Recently on a remarkable trip to Fort Benning, my son Daniel said something during dinner that made heads turn. During a discussion on leadership and integrity standards that leaders should follow, he raised his hand; he had something to say. In front of our hosts and my parents, he set a clear and unambiguous standard for his dad's behavior. It was a very simple sentence. "My dad always tells the truth." It's a sentence that has changed my life; it was a sentence that eliminated any room for compromise. It is a sentence that is so simple but means so much. Wow, what a powerful and challenging sentence. Daniel, thank you; I will do everything in my power to behave in a way that will continue to earn your trust.

SURVIVAL JOURNAL—JULY 21, 2009

Rich Versus Wealthy

Last Sunday was interesting. It was a day for Daniel and me. While it took us several hours to get out of the house, we finally went exploring. Daniel didn't know the reason for our exploration, but he got into the car with Fudge, and off we went. An hour or so later, we reached our destination, Jenny Lake and the rocks. Daniel went "bouldering" and rock climbing (clarifying for my family members that the rocks were about 3 feet high). Watching Daniel explore the lake, the rocks, and the boulders reminded me of the trips we took with my grandfather to Bowman Lake, one of the most picturesque places that I have seen. It also reminded me of how wealthy I am.

In the fall of 1975 when I met Ray Daniel. I can still visualize our first meeting. It was in the early fall of my senior year at the University of Florida. We met in the middle of a street. He was the guardian of several children who lived on the street across from me, and he was there visiting.

As a confirmed bachelor, he became the guardian of the family that lived across the street from me after both the father and mother died. During his late 30's (boy was he old), he was raising three children. Two teenagers and the youngest child, an eight-year-old boy. None of them were his. He was a wonderful man who gave and gave. In 1975 I didn't understand what made Ray wealthy. I do today.

As I grew to know Ray, I grew to respect his wisdom and the wisdom of his black lab, Sheba. He always seemed to want to listen to me, and Sheba always needed a pet. For some reason, Ray always had time to talk with me. No matter what the question or issue I faced, he seemed to understand what I was facing.

Over the first few months, we had numerous discussions about our families. He told me about his father, who was a sharecropper in Haynes City, Florida, and I told him about mine.

One day we discussed money. I had always wanted to be wealthy. At the time, I didn't know the difference between rich and wealthy, but I was about to learn. I wanted to know how he had been so successful, how he became wealthy. I asked him who was the wealthiest person he knew. He said, "Do you mean wealthy or rich?" I didn't understand. So, I then asked who the richest person was that he knew and who was the wealthiest.

He told me that the richest person wasn't that interesting but that the wealthiest person was his father. Once again, I said I didn't understand; his father was a sharecropper; how in the world could he be the wealthiest person that Ray knew? Ray told me that over 2,000 people had come to his funeral in the small town of Haines City, Florida when he died. He asked me to imagine how a sharecropper had touched that many lives. He then told me that his father did so by treating people the way he wanted to be treated, by simply following that golden rule. It was a very powerful message. It's amazing how much wealth can be created by following such a simple rule.

I often think about Ray and how much he means to me. As I've said before, you are never gone if your teachings live in the hearts and minds of others. Ray and his beloved lab passed away a few years ago. Boy, I miss him. And Sheba too. God bless you both; you both taught me so much.

November 14, 2009—What a News Day

I didn't receive the news on my biopsies Friday, and that's wonderful. Assuming that no news on Friday the 13th is wonderful news. It's all about attitude, right? So, I am looking forward to another weekend where I won't have to worry about or celebrate the results of the tests. You may be thinking I am manufacturing a positive attitude; it's a lot more than that.

You may be asking how I can think it's a wonderful day when I have to wait on tests. How could having to deal with cancer and biopsies be good news? Well, consider the alternatives. I could be a Dogs fan and dealing with cancer, but I'm not; I'm a Gator, and the Gators are currently 10-0. When I was in college, the news was the Gators lost games 10-0, had a losing record and had to play the Dogs in Jacksonville. Oh no. The fact that the Gators are 10-0, and they beat the Dogs is great news. A person can only have so many burdens, and cancer is not the one that would bother me if I were a Dog fan.

On a more serious note, going through this process has been very trying, but I believe that the future is what you make it. Furthermore, I am constantly reminded of one of my favorite phrases: "We must all give up hope for a better yesterday." So, what am I going to do tomorrow?

What I am doing is planning what I will be doing next. I am planning on my trip to Everest next May and finding some friends to go with me. Drs Foss, Kaplan, English, and Owens, please don't get in my way. Starting December 14th, I am going to start getting ready for LOTOJA 2010. For those unfamiliar, the Logan to Jackson bike race is 200 miles long. I am planning for our team to be on the podium after averaging 27 MPH. I am planning on how to build a great business. I am planning on becoming a better dad and husband. I am planning on how to move on. It's something that I hope I can do with dignity and with your support. Thanks, folks

Glenn

BAITING THE DOG

Lessons in Trust

Security is a foundational element. When you are not secure, it is very difficult to make good decisions. Likewise, when you are secure, you have fewer reasons not to make good decisions. I feel most secure when I am at home with my dog, Gator. He is a wonderful golden retriever with all the positive attributes of a golden. Every time I come home, Gator wags his tail, runs in circles, and eventually lies down at my right foot. He is the most loyal animal that I can imagine. He exhibits unconditional love, and it is mutual.

One of the things that I enjoy is coming home, drinking a glass of wine, and grilling a steak. That said, if I have the time to grill a steak, what do you think will happen if I leave the room with the steak on the counter? Everyone knows the answer to that simple question: Gator will immediately climb up on the counter and devour the steak. Heck, Gator has even eaten a chocolate pound cake that my former mother- in-law made for my ex-wife (more about that later, by the way). So, we know that there are circumstances where it's impossible to prudently trust an animal, even one that exhibits unconditional love. So, why do we trust people that we don't know well, much less individuals who we haven't known for a very long time?

If you put together my observations about Sylvia, Mr. Hodgson, and Gator, you may identify a technique that I call "Bait the Dog." This is a technique where I hope to test a person or an organization to see if I can trust them. As I stated at the beginning of this section, it is virtually impossible to trust an organization. However, there are people whom you can trust. So why not test them? The way I do this is by leaving a steak on the counter, so to speak, thereby "Baiting the Dog." You can do this by asking questions that you know the answer to, leaving money on the table, seeing if they cheat on their family, seeing if they cheat at golf, or any one of the innumerable, simple tests that can reveal their character. A well-known and very successful car dealership group uses this technique by leaving money in a car to see if a new technician takes the money while the car is in for service. If they do, they are fired. It is that simple.

Develop trust that is well founded. Don't just blindly trust someone; make a conscious, deliberate decision to trust. Make a decision that is based on facts, on observed behavior. It is the most liberating decision that you can make. By using this technique, you will start to really trust individuals. It will be the start of a series of relationships that will provide you with a secure environment that is built on a foundation of well-founded trust.

The Hodgson Test

When I was a very young lawyer, I needed to find out about a person's character. I had a mentor, Mr. Dan Hodgson, who, to this day, I believe is one the best judges of individuals, their capabilities, and their character. So, as the young lawyer, I went into Mr. Hodgson's office and asked him if he knew Mr. X. Mr. Hodgson told me sure. I then asked him how long he had known Mr. X, and Mr. Hodgson said that he had known him for more than 30 years. I then asked Mr. Hodgson, "Do you trust him; is he a man of character?" Mr. Hodgson said he didn't know anything about his character. Incredulous, I said how well do you know him? Mr. Hodgson said he and his wife had dined with Mr. X and his wife monthly for the past 30 years and that he talked to Mr. X several times each week. His answers didn't make any sense to me, so I then asked Mr. Hodgson how he could have interacted with someone that often over that many years and not know whether he could trust the person. Mr. Hodgson then looked at me with a puzzled look on his face. He seemed to be thinking. I thought this young man was smart, but I was beginning to doubt. He then provided me with a rule that is one of the foundational elements of my business life. It's a simple but very valuable axiom:

"You never know anything about a person's character until you see what they do when a lot of money is at risk."

SURVIVAL JOURNAL—
DECEMBER 1, 2009–SEPTEMBER 29, 2011

This week is another week at Yale, and I can't wait to see my friends up north. I have a PET Scan scheduled at five on Tuesday, so that means no food or caffeine after 11 a.m. On Wednesday, I meet with the Docs and vampires in the morning. By the way, that's my term of endearment. I love my vampires. I should have some information on my biopsies and the PET Scan by the middle of the afternoon.

* * *

It's Thanksgiving Sunday, and I am on my way back east after spending the week with my wife, Daniel, and Jerry (my mother-in-law). I loved the time that I spent with them. I can't get enough time with Daniel, Fudge, and Banjo. By the way, Fudge and Banjo now seem to get along, and Fudge is being permitted to spend the night in Daniel's room. I know that Fudge will hug him in the middle of the night. That couldn't be better.

I have a lot to be thankful for, and I still believe that almost everyone in the world would trade places with me. Want examples? Well, I am 55, and both of my parents are still alive and are happily married after more than 60 years.

Every time I talk to Dad, he tells me about his golf game and what's new. Mom loves walking, going to church, and playing with her great-grandchildren. What could be better? I have three wonderful children. Beth is as close to actualizing her dreams as any person I know. She is working with a startup fashion company and is as happy as I have seen her in years. The startup has a lot of promise, but the most important item is that Beth is passionate about what she is doing. Jay is in a similar position. She is a junior at Florida, where she loves working with athletes. She is passionate about her chosen profession. While it may take about ten years to complete her education, we will continue to support her as long as she is progressing and is passionate about what she is doing.

Then there is Daniel. This week he explained to me that he needs four different types of snowboards. Each type serves a different function, and as a "professional snowboarder," he has to have the right equipment. He then explained his new math system, which I believe the school understands, but I don't. Finally, he explained that he didn't want anything for Christmas because Christmas is about giving and not receiving. Boy, he made his dad proud.

As you can see, I am "wealthy" and have a lot to be thankful for. My dream in life and what I pray for is that I have children that are happy, healthy, and wise. Because if they are, they too will be wealthy. I believe that my children are on their way to achieving my dream.

Finally, there is my wife. Sunday, she gave me a kiss at the airport when I left. That little kiss means the world to me. I don't think most of us understand how a little thing like a kiss from your spouse or child will lighten your load.

What I have learned is that the simple things in life, a kiss from your wife, a passionate child, and healthy parents are the most important things in your life. Thanks for listening.

Glenn

January 6, 2010

While I know that I am still searching for my destination, I am very nervous about what Dr. Foss confirmed today. After talking to her, I have some concept about what the rest of the year will hold. It seems like I am a 2LT again. Someone else has told me that I am going on a patrol and the route that I will have to take. However, unlike those days, I will be able to determine my final destination.

I worked on different journal entries anticipating what I would find out today. Whether I start taking Ontak or not is what I was focusing on. But the more I wrote, the more I came to understand that life isn't about the next medical treatment or the next deal; it's about your family, friends, and environment. Those are the things that are important. They are the places where you can make a difference. Whether it's providing an example for your children to emulate or serving each other, you can make a difference. My daughters made a difference in my life on Christmas. I still can't get over their thought, diligence, and creativity. You see, they set an example for me to follow.

Here is the news. Effective today I went on four new prescriptions and starting January 12, 2010, I will be on an IV cocktail for a while. I am going to take my initial treatment at Yale because they have extensive experience with this regimen. Once I see how it goes, I will make a decision about whether I will take future treatments at Yale, Gainesville, or Atlanta. I am not comfortable getting the IVs in Jackson because I don't feel that they have a real cardiac ICU. Yea, that's one of the remotely possible but easily manageable side effects. Please remember that lawyers write these disclaimers; that's comforting, isn't it? I wonder how much unnecessary stress our legal system causes patients in America.

While the results and my prognosis may seem important at this instant, they really aren't that important. While I have a lot of time left on this planet, and I mean a lot of time, none of us are here all that long. But we can and should make a difference. No matter what you are facing, you have a chance to set an example for others to follow. We can change the lives of others in a meaningful way by just setting a good example. It doesn't cost money or time; it's just how you try to live your life. I hope that I don't roll around in self-pity or make my disease a defining part of my life, but I might. If I do, please remind me of my need to set a positive example and to climb mountains. Whether it's Everest or another mountain, I will find a mountain to climb. You see, I am a climber.

So it was back to Yale today, and the news is that I will be tethered to a pole for a while, and yes, it's ok to laugh at the thought. While I am not laughing right now, it's important that you do so; it's important to me that you laugh at the concept. If you laugh, it will help me climb. Your laughter will help me a lot, more than you could ever imagine.

So I have found another mountain to climb. Let's call it Mount Yale. It's not that tall of a mountain to climb. It's only two flights of stairs, not Everest's 29,035 feet, but it will still be a challenge. It doesn't take 4 or 5 weeks away from your family and friends to conquer. It takes three days to conquer, and you get to conquer this mountain every 21 days. With a little help from my friends and family, I will climb this small hill. You see, I am trying to learn, trying to think about what I can do to be the best example for Beth, Jay, Daniel, and my friends. They are what is important, and I will try never to forget that.

By the way, I hope to go to Advance Camp next year, and for some reason, I believe that Everest will still be there. We will climb that mountain together.

January 21, 2010—Happy Anniversary

It was one year ago today that I received The CALL. The best thing that has happened this year has been my realization that I have so many friends who care about me. I really can't believe that you all have been so supportive. I feel that I am one of the luckiest people in the world. Thank you. Things have changed in a year. I can't go back out to Jackson and ski with Daniel, but that's my fault. I would have been able to if I had used the training wheels George provided or if I didn't have cancer, but that's not the case. I miss Daniel more than you can imagine. I don't get to see him enough, and the treatment is making that worse. While he is in a wonderful school and environment, I wish I could have dinner with him most nights, but that's not going to happen for now.

It's been an interesting week. I finished the first regimen last Thursday and felt pretty good. I was amazed, and then Friday happened. I flew out to Jackson for the weekend. I was looking forward to seeing Daniel and pursuing the Pinewood Derby crown. (He finished 3rd)

On the way, I started feeling bloated and very tired. The longer I was on the plane, the worse I felt. Well, it turns out that I gained 24 pounds last week, yes, last week. One of our new clients owns dairies, and I believe that he would like to find out how to fatten his cows the way I fattened. Just joking; he operates organic dairies.

I contacted the docs, and when they asked how I felt, I told them I felt like Jabba the Hut trying to get into a ballet dancer's outfit. It just doesn't work. They gave me a prescription for a diuretic called Lasix, and as of Thursday, it hadn't done anything. Oh well, I always liked Star Wars, and I will watch the movie again; I want to find out what Jabba wore.

On Thursday, I went back to Yale. While there, I got to meet with my doctor and can't believe how reassuring she was. She told me that the weight gain is a reflection of one of the side effects called capillary leak syndrome. According to my docs, my reaction isn't that bad and will reverse itself quickly. She also said this reaction normally only happens after the first infusion session. Atop this, I received additional good news; Dr. Foss said that my initial reaction to Ontak looked great. She also said that my skin looked better and told me that the allergic reaction to Ontak seemed to be dissipating.

On Thursday, I felt like they couldn't do anything to get this weight off. I was wrong. I just got off of the scales and have dropped 8 pounds since Thursday. That's about 1/3 of the weight that I need to lose. I believe that I will get the rest of the weight off in the next few weeks. I am working on it, and I will make it happen.

Next week, I am at Yale on Tuesday and am scheduled to return for a three-day infusion the following week. I hope that the docs will let me keep that schedule because it will mean that I am past a lot of the side effects and that the regimen is helping. Thanks for listening.

Glenn

January 31st

It's back to Yale for the second round on Ontak. It seems like Jabba left sometime last week, and I really hope he doesn't come back. The ballet outfits seem to fit a little better, but I hope that I don't have to wear them in public, or at least not at the gym. My total weight gain was about 24 pounds, and I have lost 16 of them. So, I am on an exercise and fruit program; I miss the biscuits and gravy.

April 12, 2010—PPP Time (Pole, PET, & Port)

I am on my way back to Yale. Today will be interesting. I report in early for the installation of the port. One of the synonyms for a port is haven. Some days it seems like Yale is turning into my haven. It's turning into a safe place for me, a wonderful place where I am protected. It's a place where a wonderful group of people is working diligently to cure me. I wonder if that's why they call the city New Haven.

After they install the port, I am getting my fifth PET Scan. I won't get the results until Wednesday. The waiting is so much fun. On Tuesday, I am getting plugged in for another round of chemo. Another three days of the cocktails without getting a buzz.

Oddly, a client has decided to meet with me in New Haven tomorrow. Can you imagine traveling to New Haven to meet with me at the cancer center? Go figure. Perhaps they think I will be more focused on them because I am tethered to a pole. Not a bad strategy.

August 7, 2010—Medical Update

About six weeks ago, I was told that I would be on Ontak (IV Chemo) for an indefinite period. That will probably mean three days of Chemo every two or three weeks indefinitely. It seems to control one part of the disease, and I am tolerating it very well. Last week I was told that they were going to prescribe a new additional

Chemo Drug, Zolinza. To quote the company, "Zolinza is used in patients when the CTCL gets worse, does not go away, or comes back after treatment with other medications." In other words, it's used after recurrent failure of other treatments.

What does that mean? Really, nothing. It's just another document written by lawyers. They have to write them; it's important. That said, I believe that I am doing well, and this is just another protocol. Over the next few years, I will participate in a lot of protocols. As I said last year, it's just another cocktail. I am learning to love Yale cocktails. Yale- tails as they may become.

* * *

I started Zolinza—in addition to the IV and other drugs— about ten days ago. Today they suggested that we will double the dosage of the drug over the next ten days. Well, for the first time, I believe that they got the side effects correct, and it is possible to be exhausted, constipated, nauseous, and have diarrhea during the same day; go figure. I hope that I find the excessive weight loss side effect and lose some of the other ones.

January 13, 2011

There are a lot of reasons that I haven't written, but I won't go into them other than to say I lost Gator at the end of last year. It seems like I lost a lot last year. It might seem like too much emotional stuff. That said, I am going to start writing again.

Today I finished my first year of IV chemotherapy. 2011 looks like another year of IV chemotherapy every three weeks and oral chemotherapy each day. They have advised me that there is no end in sight for the IV protocol. At least the protocol is a regular part of my life now. At least I know what to expect.

2010 was an amazing year. I have had so many great things happen, and then there were the other things to deal with. Most importantly, 2010 was a great year for me as a father. I got to spend more time with Daniel, Beth, and Jay than I ever expected. I got to witness Daniel seeing his first shuttle launch, going to Ft. Benning, and "earning" his jump wings. His trip to West Point, and finally, his trip to Rome. They were all good for him and me too.

Beth is doing great in NY and got a wonderful promotion at the end of the year. Jay is flourishing at UF. I can't imagine how she could be doing better. They both have been a great help to me. The holiday season was almost perfect, with my three children and my parents spending time together as a family. It was a wonderful time.

Next week I will be moving out of Harris Trail and into a new home. I can't wait for that period of my life to be over. I hope that I can quickly settle into the new home.

August 13, 2011—The 31st Month

First, there was The Call; then there was the ACL; then the start of chemo, a bike wreck which broke my collar bone in September 2009 (I don't remember much about it but I hit something and woke up in the ambulance); the January 2010 start of IV Chemo, the changes in my personal and professional life; and finally, the events of the past week.

I have always anticipated unexpected events in my life, whether they are business-related or personal. You see an issue, and you develop a plan, a solution. To quote Beth, a wambulance isn't needed. As you travel through medical issues, if you pay attention and do a modicum of research, you should be able to anticipate most issues and develop workable solutions. Well, this week, I was surprised. I try to constantly remind myself of all the positive aspects of my life. That said, it doesn't mean you can't be surprised. I went to Yale for some tests based on a neuropathy issue that I was facing. They were going to run an MRI on my spine, nothing big, just another MRI to see if they could identify the cause of the issue. I was told that the neuropathy could be caused by one of several things: (i) compression of the spine as a result of the bike wreck, (ii) a side effect of the chemo, and (iii) the remote possibility that it could be MS. Well that's a few issues that can distract you for a few minutes. I had the MRI on Wednesday, and the initial, incomplete results showed nothing. I got a good night's sleep on Wednesday.

The next morning, I met with my new best friend, a Neuro-Oncologist, Dr. Kevin Becker. The assessment lasted 2 hours. A world-class Md. spent two hours with me. Once again, I should have anticipated some news, but I didn't. Well, the news is that I have a small but treatable tumor on my spine. What?

Dr. Becker continued, "It may or may not be cancerous; we need to conduct additional tests, a spinal tap to see if the cancer has migrated into the spinal fluid, a nerve connection study, blood work, genetic testing, and possibly an additional MRI. We will not have the test results until about August 20th, but we are going to the tumor board tomorrow.

I have total confidence in everyone at Yale. They are world-class professionals and very nice, caring people. Dr. Becker is the newest member of the team. He was so reassuring. He took the time to explain everything. He told me that assuming the tumor is cancer-related—and it may not be—that it would be imminently treatable. But we needed to wait for the test results to see if additional tests were needed and then develop a treatment plan.

I didn't know if I was going to write about these developments. But I felt that I needed to let a few people know what was going on. I will be back on Ontak on September sixth. I am having the nerve study on the Eight. So, the first week of the college football season will be interesting. I hope it's not interesting for the Gators.

This posting is a long way of saying that I don't know what's going on. I appreciate the support that you all give me. I may have just written an over-alarmist posting, and if I have, I want all of you to abuse me after I post the results in about three to four weeks. If I haven't been alarmist, then I want all of us to celebrate every day. We should focus on the fact that we have great friends and great families, we live in a great country, and virtually everyone in the world would trade places with all of us. Go Gators.

Glenn

September 6, 2011—W&W—The Transition of Coming to Terms with Cancer

Over the years, a few of my friends have said that I didn't understand what they told me. When that happened, I tried, I really tried to listen to them. But sometimes, you only hear part of the conversation. Well, I now know that happens when I am at Yale.

On my last visit, I was told about the tumors on my spine. I heard that they were several centimeters. They weren't. They were several millimeters. Just a small difference. But the diagnosis was correct, I have a few very small tumors, and it's in the spinal membrane.

When I received the initial report on the spinal tumors, I was told that the spinal fluid was clear. That was great news. But that news has changed. The tests indicated that there is a very small amount of cancer in the spinal fluid.

So, what happens now? What we are doing is called watching and waiting (W&W).

It feels like putting your head in a guillotine and waiting for someone to cut the rope. In reality, it's not like that. The reason you are W&W is that the problem isn't that bad. So, you wait to see if it gets worse. If it gets worse, what happens? The doctors told me that the tumor board would recommend radiation. It would be a 10-day process. That means ten days of radiation, but they believe that this would solve the problem.

That's not bad. Ten days of exhaustion and weight loss, then it's over. To my friends who went through Ranger School or Q, they know ten days is nothing. Ten days and I would be able to swing my golf clubs again. Ten days to a 30-inch waistline. That would be a wonderful result. We can all put up with ten days of anything if we believe that there is a good result coming.

I will be back at Yale in 19 days for another MRI. We will find out if the little thing has grown. If the tumor has grown, then we know what will happen. If the tumor hasn't grown, then we W&W.

September 29, 2011

The great news is that the spinal tumors have not grown at all, and the news gets better from there. I was originally scheduled to have an MRI every three weeks. They are so confident with the results that the follow-up MRIs will be every six weeks. Follow-up spinal taps will probably be on the same schedule. So, it will now be a process of wondering and worrying as we watch how this develops over the next year.

Last night they did a brain MRI with contrast. It wasn't a scheduled MRI, but the neuropathy is getting worse, and they are looking for causes and want to rule out any brain involvement with the lymphoma. The great news is that there is no evidence of tumors in the brain.

One of the positive pieces of information is that my history of long-distance running and cycling has provided significant leg strength. They told me if I weighed a lot more or hadn't exercised most of my life, I would be on either a cane or a walker by now. While it appears that the neuropathy is getting worse, I will exercise daily, so that doesn't happen. So, to all my friends, please work out. The benefits are not always apparent, but they are there. Also, each of you is authorized to berate me about working out every day. Please do so.

In late December 2009, a major change in my treatment protocol was necessary. My treatment started by taking 4 Targretin (Chemo) pills a day. After a few months, my doctor required me to increase the number of Targretin pills to six pills a day and then to eight. When we didn't get adequate results with the maximum number of Targretin pills daily, we had to try another treatment protocol. In the mid-fall, they prescribed methotrexate as an alternate Chemo protocol which also failed to be effective. Methotrexate seemed to make the cancer worse. So, my doctor decided I had to start IV Chemo in mid-December.

Starting in January 2010, I traveled to Yale every three weeks for three days of IV Chemo. Initially, I didn't know what to expect. It started as a routine three and three. Go to the Atlanta airport, park my car, get in the security line, go through TSA's security screening, and then get on the plane to New Haven. Drive to the hospital, get my blood work, start three days of Chemo, and then fly home. After a few months, the nurses started having problems finding a blood vessel to connect the IV. After two sessions like this, they decided that I needed a port. After discussing it with me, we decided to install the port on my next visit. It's easy to discuss this now, but my anxiety level was rising at the time. I didn't want a port. I always felt I could leave my cancer in New Haven, but this was different; it initially made me think I would be taking cancer with me.

On my next trip to Yale, I had one of the most amazing encounters I have had. I stood in the security line, being as patient as possible, dealing with my anxiety about the pending port surgery. After around ten minutes, the lady behind me asked me if I was ill. I thought it was a weird question. "I am fine." She persisted, and I finally admitted that I was on my way to Yale for another round of IV Chemo.

Upon hearing my answer, she said that I shouldn't be afraid. I didn't know how to react to that statement. Before I responded, she took a necklace from around her neck and put it on me. I had to move forward in the security line, so I turned around and walked forward. I then turned back to thank the lady, but she wasn't there. I asked the other people in the line if they had seen her but they all said the same thing. Who? What lady? She had just disappeared.

After I got through security, I looked at the necklace, and it had a medallion on it, and it reflected the image of the "Our Lady of Perpetual Help." Since the lady placed the necklace on me, it has only come off during surgery. I don't understand why she placed it on me. However, it has comforted me ever since during my cancer journey.

I have thought about my necklace a lot during the past decade. Recently a friend had a birthday dinner, and it turns out that most of the individuals there were Catholic. As an icebreaker, the honoree asked everyone to tell a story about one of the most unique events in their life. When it was my time to speak, I told this story. The reactions were intense. Some said an Earth Angel had visited me; most agreed that it was some sort of angelic visitation. I don't know what to call the encounter, but the necklace has comforted me for over a decade and will be around my neck for the rest of my life. Whatever the explanation, I know this act of kindness has changed my life, and I will be eternally grateful.

CANCER SET ME FREE

My Mental Approach to Survival

"When you die, it's going to be from something you love doing and not from cancer."

This was a quote from a friend of mine. She said, "I'm sure that will happen for you; that will be kicking cancer's ass." That's an important part of my formula.

Leaving Cancer Behind

What Happens at the cancer center stays at the cancer center. I came to this realization early on in my fight. During my 14+ years of chemo, I travel to Yale Medical School's Smilow Cancer Center every three or four weeks for my IV chemo infusions. When I lived in Atlanta, it wasn't that hard a trip. Now that I live in Wyoming, the travel adds a day to each treatment.

My IV chemo started out as three days of IV every three weeks, then over time dropped to one day every four weeks, and now it has increased to three days of infusions every four weeks, and it looks like we may have go to five days every three weeks.

One of my fundamental philosophies is that I leave cancer in New Haven; I leave it at Yale Cancer Center; cancer doesn't go with me. When I leave Connecticut, I'm able to restart and continue living my life. Following my passions, spending time with family and friends, playing golf, and pursuing the perfect picture. It's like I put cancer in a box and put it on a shelf at Smilow Cancer Center. While I retain responsibility for following all protocols, like taking about 50 pills a day those are just mechanical actions. I won't let cancer define me and I don't worry about it because it's in New Haven.

Cancer Tax

People always ask me how I do what I do. I tell them I don't understand the question. What else am I supposed to do. The questions seem to focus on one of two things, First how do you feel. Second, how can you spend that much time on your treatments. The key is how you treat the time tax and that's what it is.

While the first six months after my diagnosis were filled with fear, today, cancer is just kind of like a tax. There are all sorts of ways of looking at the time I spend on my treatments. The way I look at it is I still have a better way of life than most people. Since we don't have state income tax in Wyoming, I'm better off than most New Yorkers. I take chemo every day, but I don't lose anything because the cocktail works well. I lose three or more days a month, but if you look at that, that's just a little over 10% of the month, and most folks in New York pay more than 10% in taxes. So, my time tax of having to go to the hospital, getting on

Glenn Sturm

a plane, getting stuck with a needle, and not feeling perfect for a day or so after the infusion is okay. Most people don't feel perfect every day of the month.

Finding Passion

So, how do you live a life like this? You find passion. Before this period, my life was deals, work, family, and relationships—probably in that order. That's not necessarily a good thing. But today, my passion is about a lot of things. It's about doing good for others. One of my daily objectives is to put a smile on someone's face every day. It's a simple objective but it brings a lot of joy to me.

One of my principal passions is photography. Some folks actually think that I'm pretty good at photography. My photography, which I'm completely enamored with, is so important because it helps others. My passion for my photography is exploding.

So how passionate am I about my photography? When you walk in the front door of my house now, you'll see five Pelican cases, three other cases and a duffel bag ready to go. That's all the camera equipment I'm currently using because if there's something that I see or hear is available, I drop everything, load the truck, and go. I guess that comes from being a boy scout all those years ago. One of the first things they teach you is to be prepared.

A Team

Finding my passion for photography filled a void in my life. Sometimes it's too hard to do things that include others. Do you have days where you just want to be left alone to be in peace? It can be more efficient to do things alone; you don't have to build consensus. You can make decisions by yourself, without the input from others. But the problem with those four sentences is that they leave missing pieces. How do you feed your soul, your intellect, your creativity? How are you challenged? Also, a brain trust of one makes for a lesser product.

You should look at how Industrial Light and Magic was formed to create Star Wars by George Lucas. If you do, you will see that it took the collaboration of all those minds that came together to make something truly game changing. Without them, it would all have stayed in George's head.

I could have gone it alone with photography, but to be on a project like shooting eclipses changes things. For example, I have a production artist who is also a wonderful photographer. We couldn't be more different. Brit is amazing. I have learned a lot from her, her husband, and their family. When you see the book on eclipses, know that it wouldn't have happened without our team. While I take pictures of bears and other wildlife, they wouldn't be the same without her postproduction skills.

I had family members here on a recent weekend, and we went out to dinner. My daughter was shocked by how many people knew me and liked me. I told my daughter at the end, "I don't know the names of 3/4 of those people who know me." The funniest thing is when I'm in town or having dinner somewhere, five out of six times, people recognize my name. They'll say, "oh, you're the photographer." It's so different from being the lawyer, the army officer, the commander, or the dad. But now I'm the photographer.

One of the interesting things about my work is I don't sign the front of the pictures. That's because I didn't create the scene. I took a picture of it. It may be a good and unique picture, but I don't want to take away from it by putting my name on it. I sign the back of it and put a hologram on it to protect the intellectual property long term, but the image remains intact.

When you go to our local hospital you will see around 40 of my images. They were all a gift. Remember my goal to put a smile on someone's face each day. People are always telling me that they saw one of my pictures and are smiling when they tell me. I am too.

Listen Up and Do It Now

The Art of Execution and Actively Listening

I've got a phrase, "follow your heart and passion."

My Grandpa, my mom's dad, was a successful businessman. He was a wildcatter on top of starting an oilfield services company, but he got sick in his early 50s, and he sold his principal business. However, he continued to live and grow.

I loved my grandpa. He was a total straight shooter. One day I met with him and asked him if I should leave my job and go to law school. He told me, "Don't be on your death bed wishing you had done something. Do it and do it now, and you'll do fine.

My father was a career Army officer. His favorite expression that he drilled into me every day was: Decision by indecision is the worst decision of all. He said not making a decision is, in fact, making a decision. People will respect you as a leader if you do something. Sitting on the sidelines and letting circumstances dictate the outcome is not acceptable.

The acknowledgments of people and what they did for me are important. I had two older gentlemen who were mentors for most of my business life. One was Daniel Hodson, and the other one was Ray Daniel. So, it was kind of important that my son, when I had one, be named Daniel.

Ray had the most important phrase. When I was young, he once said to me, "Glenn, you're very smart, and you're almost always correct, but you need to learn how to listen. You need to learn how to get others to do things because they want to do them, not because you told them to do them." He taught me that listening is the most important business skill that you can have.

He taught me active listening as well as many other important skills and lessons. He was so important in my life. When I was a lawyer, he was my first client. My first project for him was the acquisition of a failing financial institution.

He hired my firm and me before I got my bar results. The engagement letter was signed as "candidate for admission to the bar." The firm didn't believe me; they couldn't believe that a very successful businessman would hire a very recent law school graduate. The office's managing partner told me to go get a $10,000 check and get this letter signed, and we will take the client. I went down and saw Ray; he wrote me a check for $10,000, signed the letter, and I showed up back in Atlanta with check and document in hand. The firm didn't know what to do because I was a first-year lawyer with his own clients.

Ray had a lot of confidence in me, and it was contagious. His confidence in me made me confident in myself. This is one of the many reasons why I made partner so soon out of law school. I had more clients than a lot of the partners in the firm when I was an associate. Ray's confidence in me also made me work harder. I couldn't let him down by missing something. It made me a better man.

Mr. Hodson was the managing partner for around three decades at one of the largest law firms in the country. Before Dan went home to hospice, he had an office next to me in every building we occupied. Whenever I had a problem, I could go and ask him about it. I didn't always do what he said, but his insight was invaluable. Finding people in your life that are smart and people whom you trust will change your future. The key is when you find them, listen to them. You may not always agree with them, but you will have that recourse that will change the velocity and direction of your life. It certainly did mine.

Loyalty is a two-way street. Both wonderful gentlemen taught me that. Loyalty is earned, trust is earned, and both are easily lost.

When I was one of the leaders of the law firm, we had five people who made all the decisions. I was not always popular because my billing rates were materially higher than others, and I shared credit for everything. Not all the other leaders in the firm shared credit. However, there was another partner who was better at sharing than me. Over the firm's duration, he is probably the most successful partner in the firm. He reminds me of the wonderful philosophical statement: It's amazing what you can build when you don't worry about who gets the credit.

In active listening, you don't mirror what somebody says. If someone says, "the dog is brown," you could reply, "oh, that's a brown dog." That's a good start but you can do better. In active listening, one could say, "he really must love dogs to notice that color." You hear their idea, you listen to their idea, and you make sure they know that you've heard the idea. Then, you may add something to the idea after showing that you have given it thought. It's an important technique, and people who do that have a lot easier job leading.

Leading

My dad always told me that when you assign a job to somebody, you never tell them how to do it. You will be surprised by their creativity, and you will learn from people who do things a different way. That's critical because it empowers the person that's working for you; it shows them respect. In the end, they will be more passionate about what they do when you let them do it their way.

When you put down rules on how to do everything, people may become rebellious or resentful. When you show them respect you may learn something, and it goes a long way to developing loyalty.

There's something called the ODA Mission Planning Guide. ODA stands for Operational Detachment Alpha, which is one of the smallest units in the Green Berets. The guide outlines how to plan a mission. It is one of the best business planning tools I've ever seen. You can  scan the code above to read the document on my website. If you apply the guide's tools to business issues, I believe you obtain better processes and business results. But one of the things about this process is that the plans are built from the bottom up, not top down. You can't be successful with this leadership technique unless you can really understand the people. Just like Ray Daniel told me, you've got to learn how to listen.

In the Kerry/Obama democratic primary election, I think Kerry blew the election by not actively listening during the debate. Obama said something like, "we are drilling more wells now than ever," and Kerry missed a big opportunity. They're drilling more wells because the approval process takes four years. The drilling Obama was referring to was approved by Bush. I think Kerry's response should have been, "we are drilling more now than we ever have. That's because President Bush approved them, and you haven't approved anything meaningful. Every well you've got, President Bush approved." He wasn't listening. But if he had actively listened and agreed with him that we are drilling more now than ever and then added that phrase, he could have reshaped the argument showing that Obama took credit for all of Bush's work. That's a good example of not active listening. Really, it is about thinking while listening rather than just hearing the words.

Find Your Weaknesses and People Who Have Complementary Skills

There's a speech that I did about the art of building lasting companies. The key is putting people in jobs that make them successful. Look at their strengths, and when you find their weaknesses—and we all have them—you help them build a complementary team. My production artist Brittany—who ideas sometimes are as crazy as a June bug. She is so focused on the pixel level of pictures and picking the right medium to print on that some people have a hard time getting along with her. I wonder if it's because they envy her talent. You should know that I would be nearly as good as I am without her and what she has taught me. Her skills complement mine. She fills a hole in my swing.

I respect her technical skills and her proficiency, and I don't think there's anybody else in the world as good as she is at what she does. Finding relationships like that in building businesses are critical. Brittany always says that we look at everything from different sides, and she's right. My point is that I trust her to do it her way, and we always get there. It's just like my dad taught me, when you assign a job to somebody, you never tell them how to do it. You will be surprised by their creativity, and you will learn from people who do things a different way. It was worth repeating.

Problem Solving and Critical Thinking

I look at most problems in a very specific way, not being some-thing black and white. I use a decision-making process. It's a very objective method. But once I get all the objective data, I make a decision based on subjective reasoning. Some people will hold up a piece of paper and say there are two sides to anything One thing to remember is that there are not just two sides to a problem/disagreement.

There are many more ways to look at the problem. It's like a ball, not the two sides to a piece of paper. To make it more complex, there is an inside and outside of a ball. You must look at it from all perspectives. When I hand people a metaphorical ball, they rarely look on the inside. You must look from the inside too. Then, you must ask questions to see what's important to the other person. You may see the perfect answer while they are looking at the issue in a different way. For instance, they may see the problem as an electric car, and you think the problem is a Zebra. You've got to solve their electric car issue in order to get them to your Zebra. Again, active listening helps, and you may learn that the real solution is the electric car.

During my time at the law firm, if two of us on the executive committee agreed on something it normally happened. One day I told the other member that we almost always agreed if we had the same information. From then on when we disagreed, we searched for the disparity in information, and we almost always found it. It turned to be one of the best business relationships that I have ever had.

Speaking of critical thinkers and active listening, Admiral Raymond A. Spruance is a person I have studied and admired. In my life I have tried to emulate him and his leadership approach. He was a quiet man who never sought public recognition for what he accomplished. He stayed away from the press. He spent his time developing his units and the people in them. He was always studying problems and history. He would not stop studying a problem until he

had examined all aspects of the problem. For good reason he was known as the most cerebral and reserved Admiral during WWII. His biography, "A Study in Command" is a wonderful read.

Golf is a sport that you can never perfect, no matter how good you are. It took me seven years after playing again—I've been playing since I was three—to figure out how to get distance back in my drives, and I've done it. I learned a simple change from the most junior instructor at my club. It was a good use of active listening. The solution broke all the rules of what people think is the best way to get more distance. Golf is just physics and geometry, she taught me to add weight to the driver head. Same speed but more weight. More mass at the end of the pendulum with the same speed equals more distance. My swing may be a very little bit slower, it's also more accurate. The net result is the ball goes further because I have more mass in the club head which results in more efficiency. Some of the pros have said they can't believe my distance or my smash factor. They're in their 30s, and I'm in my late 60s. Again, nobody could fix it for me. They thought hitting the ball 240 yards at my age was good, but now I'm hitting it over 270 regularly. The best part about it is that a friend of mine who's a better golfer than I am goes crazy that I can hit the ball so much further than he can. It's just fun.

What's important is figuring out the problem. What had I been doing that created the lackluster result? What is the solution to the problem? Finally, how do you change the process to prevent making the mistakes or having lackluster performance in the future?

Try focusing on learning about your mistakes or unacceptable performance. What did you do wrong that caused the issue? You should also celebrate your mistakes, own them. Only then will you have learned something meaningful from making a mistake. Some people call them "after-action reports" or "after-action analyses," but most people are too concerned with the right, wrong, and blame versus understanding. Only you can stop you. You can accept where you are, or you can work out how to change your state.

How Exactly did Cancer Set Me Free?

I was successful beyond my wildest expectations as a lawyer and running a public company, but there were a lot of holes. I didn't want to leave my position, but basically, I got cancer, and I had to leave the law firm. I had to stop practicing law. I loved most of the boards that I was on, and I loved my job, but when I left, I had all this time. What was I going to do with myself? I was not going to be a couch potato. I started by religiously working out six days a week in the gym and do everything the doctors told me to do. That is one of the reasons I've done so well. That wasn't enough. Cancer survival comes down to how I live and think.

I had to find something. So, I used the problem-solving lessons that I had learned. I studied my disease. I studied all my medications. I asked a lot of questions. I focused on active listening. I found things that I would never have found if I hadn't had cancer. Cancer cut me loose. It cut the strings that tied me to what I had been doing for so many years.

I found out that I really loved photography. I found out that I can be a good friend. I found out how many friends I had that I didn't know I had. It really freed me from all the shackles that I put on myself to succeed. Beyond financial success and status, where do you go? I started worrying a lot more about making the world a better place. I started focusing a lot more on helping other people. My psychiatrist would probably say that I help others almost to a fault, but when you do that, you change lives.

Helping

An example of this is when I helped my former server at my favorite breakfast joint. I noticed that Shalya was no longer working at the restaurant. I really missed her, she was always so nice to everyone. A few months after I noticed that she had left the restaurant, I was working on a project to rebuild an Alfa Spider. I needed help with the upholstery. I mentioned this to a friend, and she told me that Shayla had started an upholstery business. I got her phone number and asked her if she wanted the project. She did and did a wonderful job.

During the rebuild process I started thinking about Shalya and everything she had done to help others. I started thinking what could I do to help her build her business besides paying for the work. I had some empty space in my workshop and giving her a workshop where she could expand her business might help. I offered her the space for free and it took a while for her to accept. She is a very proud woman.

She's got a robust business today. She asked me what she could do for me. I told her that the only thing I'd ask from her in return is to do the same thing for someone down the track that I did for her. It would have been easy for me to just hire her for her services and be done with it, but it cost me very little to help her build a real business, and it had a real impact. I always am trying to find someone to help build a business and become truly independent. It is a whole pay-it-forward philosophy that I have embraced, and it puts smiles on people's faces. It also reminds me of the opportunities to help people that I missed. I'm working hard to not miss those in the future.

To date all the revenue that I have received from my photography has gone to charities to support children's health, battered shelters, and PTSD. While I can spend time on my passion which is landscape, wildlife, and astrophotography, more importantly, I am able to help others. Again, this puts a smile on people's faces, and mine too.

My point is: if I hadn't been set free from working diligently for 14 hours a day, 51 weeks a year, who knows what shape I would be in now? For the past 13.5 years, the line's been cut, and it set me free to pursue all these things that I love doing, which is to help others, and it's so rewarding. "Cancer saved my life and set me free," as a central philosophy, is a key ingredient in my attitudinal tool kit. Instead of spending energy hating or fearing cancer, I create energy for myself by being thankful for what it has given me.

SURVIVAL JOURNAL—
MARCH 15, 2012–SEPTEMBER 17, 2014

I just achieved a milestone during my recent IV Chemo treat-
ment. I have finished my 100th session of IV Chemo. Over 100
days in the infusion center, 100 days of visiting and interacting
with a wonderful group of nurses, paraprofessionals, nurse prac-
titioners, physician assistants, and doctors.

They are an amazing group of individuals who are totally sup-
portive, caring, and a wonderful group of professional friends.
Thank you, while I can't thank everyone, I want to specifically
thank Barbara, Sunshine, Mel, Malou, Lisa, Zandi, and, of course,
Dr. Foss. The journey wouldn't be what it is without you.

Now that I have made my politically correct but sincere com-
ments, I want to talk about the century. When you hear about a
century, you may think about a lot of different things that make
up a century. Some of my friends think about a 100-mile bike
race, others think about the turn of the century, while others
think about living for 100 years and, for a few crazy friends,
a 100-mile ultra-marathon. They are all milestones, a form of
accomplishment; something to measure; something to achieve.

So how are 100 IV Chemo sessions a milestone, an accomplishment, or something to achieve? Well, it beats the alternative.

The first individual I met over three years ago at Yale. He has the same form of T-Cell lymphoma that I have and has been fighting the fight for more than a decade. About seven years ago, he was told by a major cancer center that there was nothing else they could do and that he should "go home and get his personal affairs in order." That's when he went to Yale and met Dr. Foss. He was put on Ontak, and seven years later, his affairs are in order, and he is still taking Ontak every two weeks. Imagine 26 sessions a year for more than seven years. Heck, he is either close or has passed his 200th session of IV Chemo. He's, my hero.

Last fall, when the FDA took Ontak off of the market, we both developed the same type of tumors within weeks. As a result of the persistence of both of our medical teams, we were both granted "compassionate use." After getting back on Ontak, it appears that Ontak is working for both of us. He believes that the tumors aren't growing, he believes that working out regularly helps the treatment, and he knows that attitude and support are the keys to surviving, to achieving another century. He is a wonderful example to the rest of us. Let's celebrate his next century, and mine too.

August 28, 2012

I lost my father today. Dad's death was a great tragedy, and we will miss him every day of our lives, but he was still teaching me things when he was in the hospital. He had the nurses joking and laughing. He faced his adversity with a wonderful sense of humor.

I thought things were going so well with him that I kept my chemo appointment at Yale. When I left the hospital after spending every night there after the accident and through his surgery, the hospital had scheduled his transfer to a rehabilitation hospital.

You can imagine my shock when I was told during a chemo session that dad had died. I am trying to focus on the positive things that I received from my father, what he taught me and that I need to teach those lessons to others.

I have to share my favorite story about my dad. This is a story that I have heard from several of my Dad's contemporaries over the years. Just thinking about it makes me smile. After the Battle of the Bulge, Dad was going to give up his command and move to the regimental staff. You see, they didn't know what to do with a 20-year-old 1st Lieutenant Battalion Commander. He couldn't stay as a Battalion Commander; he was too junior. He couldn't go back to being a Company commander because he had already been a Battalion Commander. So, the powers dictated that Dad would move up. The powers decided that he would be the Assistant Regimental S-3, a Major's slot. Before the change of command, there was a "beer blast." party Dad was doing paperwork at his desk. Several of Dad's soldiers burst into his tent office. They insisted that Dad come join the party. Dad's Sargent Major watched the interaction for a few minutes, snickering all of the time. The Sargent Major couldn't take it any longer and started laughing so hard that he started crying. The soldiers couldn't stand the Sargent Major's behavior and asked why he was laughing. The Sargent Major asked a question. "How old do you have to be to drink?" The soldiers quickly replied 21. The Sargent Major then asked the soldiers, "how old is the Old Man?" The Sargent Major then quickly answered for them. He ain't there yet. The Sargent Major then explained that the CO, our Dad, wasn't old enough to drink. If he went to the party, he would have to enforce the rules. He told them that the "Old Man" knew that the entire organization had earned the beers, but he would not personally violate the rules and would not let violations that he saw go uncorrected. As a result, he decided not to attend his party because even though he

117

was the "Old Man," the "Old Man" wasn't old enough to drink. He was taking care of his troops; he subordinated his personal enjoyment so that his troops would benefit. That was his responsibility. That is our Dad's legacy.

Dad always showed me over the years that he was a man of character, a person whom you should trust, and a person for all of us to emulate. His behavior, in this case, showed what he always taught me. Take care of your troops. That is your first job.

February 14, 2013—I'm in 5th Grade

I can't believe it, but I am now in my fifth year of daily Chemo and my fourth year of IV Chemo. That's over 71 trips to New Haven, over 200 days in New Haven, and over 200 days being taken care of by my wonderful medical team. As the old expression goes, time flies when you're having fun.

July 16, 2013

I tend to write when I can find things to laugh about. I have recently found some things to laugh about and, upon reflection, some very positive things to talk about. I have some observations, but let's just laugh at what's been on my plate.

My Neuro-oncologist stopped by recently while I was in the hospital and told me that they believed that they finally knew why my voice was getting softer and rougher. He told me that they had identified a very small tumor on my spine that might be impacting my speech. He told me that this could be magnified when I was tired. So that's one at the top of my spine and one at the bottom. To quote military terms, it appears that the Lymphoma has its target bracketed.

August 23, 2013

I was hospitalized earlier this year because of an infection. It wasn't that bad, and I thought we had dealt with it. I was wrong. When I got to Yale on Tuesday, I had a CT scan and determined that the infection was back. So, I am now back on high-dose antibiotics for at least the next ten days and probably longer. There is a possibility that I will have to go on a prophylactic antibiotic regimen for a very long time. Hey, it's just more components to the cocktail. The other requirement is that I can't have more than 15 grams of fiber in a day. As most of you know, I was never that big on green vegetables, so now I have a legitimate reason not to eat them.

October 4, 2013

I just finished my 200th day of IV Chemo. I'm an IV Chemo double centurion. In addition, I have now completed approximately 1,675 days of taking chemo orally. It seems like my life has become a pattern; most days seem like the days in the movie Ground Hog Day. I get up, take the first set of meds, wait an hour, eat a snack, do physical therapy, take more meds, try to remember the schedule, take more meds at lunch, etc. Well, something new is going to happen now, but before I discuss that, I wanted to provide a joke.

Three professionals were discussing the nature of God. The doctor said, "The Bible states that God made Woman by taking a rib out of Man; God is obviously a surgeon." The engineer replied, "But before God made man, he created Heaven and Earth out of Chaos; this is obviously the work of a master engineer." The lawyer just smiled and said, "But who do you think created the chaos?"

Life has seemed chaotic for the past few months. The infection that we are going to attack has caused part of the chaos, but there have been other factors as well that have created uncertainty. Part of that uncertainty was eliminated when we decided that I was going to undergo surgery to eviscerate the infection. The surgery next week is the first of two surgical procedures over the next two months. The surgery this week is scheduled for between four and five hours. I've been told that while there is risk in every surgery, for the following reason, mine should be easier:

Three surgeons were discussing their favorite type of patients. The first said: "I like artists. When you cut them open, they are awash with color inside." The second doctor said: "I much prefer engineers. When you cut them open, everything is orderly and numbered." "Nonsense," said the third doctor. "The easiest are attorneys. They have only two parts, their rear end and their mouth, and those are interchangeable."

October 10, 2014

The surgery lasted approximately 3 hours. Jay was just briefed by the doctors, and the news is good. They confirmed that I am the appropriate owner of the BS Trademark because even though they saw none in me, they saw the results of almost 60 years of BS. Scan the QR to see the BS trademark in action.

September 17, 2014—The Sixth Year

It looks like it's approximately 2,025 days of oral chemo and 211 days of IV chemo. When you add travel to that amount and time in the hospital for surgery, I have spent over a year in New Haven since January of 2009.

Today was supposed to be another day of IV chemo, another of my groundhog days. Well, it didn't work out that way. When I got to the hospital, I was informed that they were going to rerun certain blood tests. So, since you know me, you know that I needed an immediate answer to the question, why? The answer to my question was that the last few tests indicated that I might be in renal failure mode. While they believed that it was controllable, they wanted to rerun the tests before they gave me chemo.

What I have never talked about before today is that this is the third time that I have had a major side effect that might be "interesting." The first one turned out to be drug-induced hepatitis. The second interesting side effect caused the multiple rounds of surgery last year. In both of those cases, my chemo was suspended temporarily, and in both cases, I ended up with additional tumors. So, as you can imagine, I am particularly focused on maintaining my chemo regimen and the remaining parts of my cocktail.

After about an hour's wait, the test results were back, and the creatinine and eGFR levels showed Stage 3B Moderate CKD renal failure. But to quote The Renal Association, "In many cases, changes in medicines or other simple changes will be enough to put things right." So, the conclusion today was no IV chemo or oral chemo until I get better blood test results. So if any of my friends see me drinking anything other than water (except one Diet Coke to go with my morning meds) or eating nuts, please feel free to abuse me. I am sure this is just another small hill to climb, but I intend to run up the hill and get this behind me so that I can get back on my chemo.

In addition, it seems that I have a six-by-seven-centimeter mass on my back. It doesn't feel like it is attached to the UFO on my spine, but they want an immediate image and biopsy of the mass. I won't know the results for several days. It's probably much ado about nothing.

LESSONS I LEARNED OVER FOURTEEN FOGGY AND DIZZYING YEARS

The reason that I started with this long war story is that it reflects the most important lesson that I have learned during my cancer battle.

If you are reading this book because you have had a similar diagnosis or somebody you know has been diagnosed, my hope is that what I have learned can be helpful to you.

How to improve your quality of life:
- Most people think that getting an incurable cancer is a bad thing, it created an opportunity for me.
- You control whether you are happy. Cancer doesn't have to define you.
- Put a smile on someone's face every day
- We must all give up hope for a better yesterday
- I believe that the world will materially improve if each of us asks ourselves the following question every day on our way home from work—What have I done today to make another person's life better or to make another person's job easier?

- Decisions by indecision is the worst decisions of all
- Only you can stop you
- Never quit never ever quit

To survive cancer for fourteen years you must learn, know, and understand:
- Your complete medical condition and how it affects your day-to-day life.
- The effects of the medicines, any possible drug interactions for the medications you take, and how they will impact your medical conditions.
- Assume that there will be drug interactions between all the medications you take. Always ask your pharmacist if the pharmacist sees any possible drug interactions. Later I will tell you never to assume things, but like always, there are exceptions to every rule.
- The changes in your test results and see if they correspond to changes in your medical conditions. Track the changes. Look at the trends.
- You may not get these reports from your hospital, but it's easy to create an excel spreadsheet.
- Challenge your doctors. Ask questions about:

  a. If there should be changes in the way your conditions are being treated.

  b. If your conditions are changing, then ask a question.

- When new medications are prescribed, read all the warnings and see if you think that they may aggravate your conditions. Again, ask your pharmacist if there are any drug interactions. Before taking any new medication, question your doctors.
- Don't just rely on what you think your medical providers are doing. Don't assume that they know the answers to these

questions. You must understand what they are doing and why they are doing it.

- Again, ask questions. I know it is difficult during the COVID period to bring someone to be with you but bring someone with you. Normally they will do a better job of remembering what was said. For some reason, they may be distracted.
- Be prepared. Almost all doctors are great and take the time to be prepared. However, you can help them provide you better care by taking the time to prepare for your meetings with them. Write down your issues and medical history and provide it to them. You will be the major beneficiary of your preparation. We are all humans with numerous distractions. I believe that Doctors make assumptions about their patients based on the information that they have. As an example, unless you tell the doctor about yourself, they won't know that you work out every day. You can have a materially positive impact on your medical future by being careful, skeptical, and thoroughly informed about yourself, your conditions, and the possible side effects of medications. Make sure you communicate this information to your doctors. Make sure you ask questions and write down the answers.

SURVIVAL JOURNAL—NOVEMBER 26, 2015–JANUARY 1, 2022

November 26, 2015

Thanksgiving again. What a perfect day to be my 2,500th- day fighting cancer. I am celebrating life. I am thankful for each day and for many other wonderful things that have happened over the past 6.8 years. There are lots of things that have been difficult; some I will talk about and others that I won't. If you remember one thing about this post, please remember to celebrate each day you are on our planet. It is a gift.

There have been a few surgeries along the way.
1. ACL Tear February 2009 the last of 6 knee surgeries
2. Rebuilding Crushed Collar Bone October 2009
3. Rebuilding Crushed Collar Bone 2 January 2010
4. Kidney Stone 1 April 2013
5. Kidney Stone 2 May 2013
6. Abdominal Surgery 1 October 2013

7. Abdominal Surgery 2 November 2013
8. Abdominal Surgery 3 April 2014
9. Abdominal Surgery 4 October 2014
10. Throat Surgery October 2015
11. Throat Surgery 2...

There are only a few things I am certain that I have learned during this journey:

First, my old favorite, "We must all give up hope for a better yesterday." Boy, isn't that the truth, and I wish I had come up with that line.

Second, I firmly believe that we determine our own future. Said another way, the future will hold what we make of it.

Finally, and most importantly, I believe that the world will materially improve if each of us asks ourselves the following question every day on our way home from work—What have I done today to make another person's life better or to make another person's job easier?

January 21, 2016—Lucky Seven

Yesterday, I finished another round of IV chemo, and today is the 7th anniversary of my diagnosis. That fateful day when I will always remember where I was—at the Atlanta airport, Gate B13 waiting for my flight to Raleigh. The Call that changed my life.

December 4, 2016

Edith Lackey Sturm—December 4, 1925 – December 4, 2016.

I received another type of one-off phone call today. My brother-in-law called and shared the very sad news that my mother had passed. I was told she passed easily; she just stopped breathing. My mom had once again made it easy on us. We will never have a problem remembering the day she passed. It was her 91st birthday.

I will miss her more than you can imagine. I was devastated that I was unable to talk with her on her birthday. I will always regret that failure.

You see, mom was always there for us, and I have work I need to do there. While growing up, dad deployed and went to war. Mom was there for breakfast, lunch, and dinner seven days a week, fifty-two weeks a year. A caring, nurturing, and continuously supportive mom.

My favorite memories as a child were of my mom doing something to support me. She always told me I was smart and that I could accomplish anything that I put my mind to. While she wasn't a pushover, she politely encouraged all of us. She imbued us with confidence. She just knew her children would be ok. She knew we would all excel at whatever we decided to pursue. She set the example with her own behavior. If you emulated mom, you would excel. That said, I was recently told that my mom said that I would either be President of the US or in jail. I am happy to say that I failed her on both accounts.

January 21, 2017—Eight Years Later

It's been 2,922 days of growing while dealing with cancer. I guess I'm counting. That said, I'm looking forward to another 15,000 days of growing while I fight the disease.

To me, it's stunning that it's been eight years. Daniel has doubled in age and height. I've lost my mom, dad, and several other members of my family. I have also lost twenty percent of my waistline and an inch of my height. I wonder if that's related. While I lost all those things, I believe I have gained more than I have lost.

I have gained insight into myself and my needs. I have learned how much I need others and how independent I am. At times I withdraw and don't communicate, especially when I have difficult things to deal with. That's not necessarily the best way to handle things, but it is how I am able to deal with difficult things like cancer. It is one of the reasons I try to work out with my physical therapists or head to the parks right after chemo to take pictures. Both of these activities help me recover from the poison that is injected into me every other week and that I take each day. That said, I love working out and going to the park to rest and take pictures. They help me grow. They teach me how to get better.

Over the past eight years, I have observed the reality shows that have invaded our television networks. They show people who intentionally place themselves in peril (while the TV cameras are watching). These days I laugh at them. I have been to a lot of those places, and they are amazing. I will acknowledge that my hotel rooms may be nicer than their tents. However, we all know that they have nothing on chemo, a 28-kilo backpack, and hiking by yourself. You see, cameras and lenses weigh a bit, but it is my lens into the world. It is amazing to me that I have discovered that I do have a left side of my brain, and when I exercise that size of my brain, I feel a lot better.

My real question is what I have missed during the past eight years. I want to know what I could have done better and how do I ensure that I can make my family, friends, fellow patients, people I meet, and the world a better place. I want to ensure that I don't miss the same things during the next eight years. That means that I will have to keep my eyes and ears open and, hopefully, my mouth shut. (Everyone knows how hard that is and will be for me.) I try to learn new things and find wonderful new people, places, and images.

January 22, 2018—My Tenth Year

The tenth year of my cancer journey starts today. I have finished nine years of continuous treatment. I am sending this journal entry while I am on my way back to Yale for another round of Romidepsin (my IV Chemo). I can't wait to get there, see my friends and get back to Atlanta as soon as possible.

I had just turned 55 when this started and have now gone through nine years of continuous chemo. While there have been highs and lows today, the highs and lows are so much higher than I could have ever imagined. I have made many new friends during the journey, from the staff at the Study Hotel, to the Delta employees in Hartford and, of course, the many doctors and staff at Smilow Cancer Center. Thanks to all of you who have helped me weather this time.

When I wrote The Call all those years ago, I didn't believe I would have nine great years. I didn't believe that I would have the quality of life that I have experienced.

September 3, 2018—The Chemover™

There is a so-called "curse" coined or embellished by Sir Austen Chamberlain in1936: "may you live an interesting life." I feel that somebody may have vexed me with such intent, having experienced my recent months.

My chemo cocktail has changed several times. About nine weeks ago, my doctors increased the IV chemo concentration 3x. I assumed that even though I had another major breakout this past week—two sessions after the IV concentration increase—that the 3x increase would be enough, but after my examination and some tests, I was told that we would be increasing the IV concentration again during my next round. In addition, I was told to double the number of Targretin pills that I take each day. The result of the first increase in the concentration in the new cocktail is an amazing increase in the side effects.

The recent cocktail has created a wonderful Chemover™ (thanks, Jack, for that wonderful job of word-smithing). I believe that during the Chemover™ recovery period, which can last a week or more, sometimes I transform into a true curmudgeon. I won't admit that I am always a curmudgeon. If you disagree, please keep that to yourself. I only hope that after the newest IV and pill regimen takes effect, the side effects won't get worse or that my "occasional" curmudgeon-like behavior doesn't amplify. On a personal note, the past eight months have been wonderful. Beth, Jay, and Daniel are doing great. Daniel is in the process of selecting his university and finishing high school. Greg and Beth's restaurant, The Anchorage, was named a semifinalist for the James Beard Best New Restaurant in the United States and had a wonderful article written about the restaurant in the New York Times. Jay just seems to enjoy her profession more and more. I am so proud of my children.

July 22, 2019—My Interesting Life Continues

It has not been a smooth year. I just wanted a quiet, uneventful year. Well, I haven't gotten my wish yet. As it stands today, so far this year, I have had six surgeries, five with general anesthesia.

It started on December 30th. I woke up, and my left eye had what looked like a sunglass lens on the lower half of my left eye. Later that day, I called my Ophthalmologist and reported the issue. She saw me Sunday morning at 9 am.

After a few minutes, she told me that she needed to refer me to a retinal surgeon. She believed I had a significant problem. I did.

The Eclipse Shoot

We just got back from Chile, where we shot the sunset eclipse on July 2, 2019. It went extremely well. Once again, we were blessed with wonderful weather. We met an exceptional group of Chileans. Everyone was wonderful. From the executive director of an observatory to the head  of the Maritime Police in Chungungo, the individuals were all engaging and helpful. We shot the eclipse on the Chilean coast at Puerto Cruz Grande, which is very close to Chungungo. The eclipse was a sunset eclipse. We were amazed by the sincerity and warmth of the individuals. Scan the code to view the image and take the 3D virtual tour of my gallery exhibit. In the gallery, you will see a copy of a photograph of the diamond ring. I took the picture at the Eclipse on July 2, 2019, in Chile. It's one of approximately 9,000 pictures taken that day from five cameras.

February 12, 2020—Twelve-Years-On

Here I am, twelve years on the journey, and I have the blessing of living to meet my first grandchild, Samuel Rowan McPhee. 8 pounds 11 ounces. Sam, Beth, and Greg and doing very well. Beth is a fantastic mother. I can't wait for Sam to get a little bit older and start telling me what I'm doing wrong. I'm sure that Aunt Jay and Uncle Daniel will provide him guidance on the matter.

January 21, 2021—Hey, Let's Have a Pandemic

At the time of diagnosis, I was 54. Daniel was 9. Jay was 22. Beth was 26 and single. Our family has since thrived. Daniel, now 20, is a COVID college student. Jay has her graduate degree and loves her profession. Beth, too, has her graduate degree and is married to Greg.

I am 67. I have been on oral chemo since March 2009 and IV chemo since January 2010. That is well over 4,000 days of oral and over 500 IV Chemo treatments. The only breaks in this process occur when I undergo surgery. Not surprisingly, I now benefit from, if not also enjoy a personal relationship with several members of the Anesthesiology department at Yale New Haven Hospital.

As I start my 13th year of dealing with cancer, I believe that I have learned a few things: It isn't cancer or chemo with which you deal each day; it's how you choose to mentally deal with having cancer that will determine how your life goes. This will be easier for some than others. That said, I believe that you shouldn't let cancer define you. I don't believe that I have let cancer define me; I am a very blessed man.

When I started this process, I aimed to create a destination and to have a great journey for however long I would get. I never expected to have 12 years. I expected to have only three, maybe four. Thank you, Dr. Foss, and your wonderful team, for this extra time. I tell everyone I know that I don't go to Yale for treatment, I go to Dr. Foss wherever she may be.

I hope that those of you who know me see that, for this "duo-decennial period," I have been "creating my destination" and celebrating each day with which I am blessed. I am honestly just trying to have fun. From watching my children develop into wonderful adults to using photography as my creative outlet, I am enjoying an interesting and wonderful journey.

January 1, 2022—So, How Am I Doing?

Generally, I am doing very well. Especially considering I am now beginning my fourteenth year on this journey. Furthermore, some sources say you aren't a geriatric until you are 80, and I'm not close to 80. So, there is no need to worry about me. I work out six out of seven days each week other than those days when I don't. Like when I'm on a plane flying to chemo or for other "good" reasons. The workouts are important for two reasons. First, they help metabolize  the chemo and other drugs that I inject into my body each day. Second, they let me continue to live a relatively active lifestyle.

I lost Blitzen and Fudge last summer to cancer. Unfortunately, they didn't have the benefit of my medical team. The newest member of the Sturm household is Lulu. She is a well-trained 6-month-old golden retriever. Please scan the code to take a look at the images in the gallery. You will see that she is a little bit spoiled.

P.S. After I wrote this post Blitzen, Jr arrived. He was born on December 25, 2021. He is now the larger of the two Goldens.

FINAL WORDS

Several years ago, I had a very serious and complicated surgery scheduled. For the first time, I was afraid. I didn't know, heck, I didn't think I was going to make it. I didn't know if I was going to wake up from the surgery. I wrote the following note to my children. Luckily it was never sent.

Let no sorrow set upon you
or your heart, for I am free.

To My Amazing Children

You, all of you, were my heart and soul. I smiled every day because of the joy each of you brought me. You see, since 2009, or was it 2010, or 2014, or maybe 2016, or was it 2019, something happened that set me free. I don't know whether it was cancer, the events of those years, or the cumulative effect of those events that finally set me free, but free I am. I have many regrets. I know I did not live up to my potential and made more mistakes than days I lived. I know that I should have done better. I wish I could erase my mistakes. I can't.

Please forgive me for my countless misgivings. I hope you believe that I deserve mercy. As you think about my life, please grant me mercy, and accept my apology for the countless mistakes I made during my life.

I hope that, on most days, I brought you joy. Every day, I wanted to put a smile on your face. I know that each of you brought me joy every day. You placed countless smiles on my face. I hope you realize the joy you brought me.

You see, cancer set me free. Once I was blessed with this disease, my burdens lifted. My eyes were opened, albeit slowly at times, but they were opened. Unlike lots of friends who died suddenly, I was given the greatest gift, TIME. Time to reflect and time to heal.

Maybe the best hill I had to climb was the difficulties I encountered with my eyes. I thought I knew myself, saw myself. I thought my eyes saw things clearly without bias or inappropriate filters. I made the mistake of "seeing things clearly." Well, after seven eye surgeries, I needed coke bottle glasses for me to see things in focus. That may have described my life because, most days, I never wore glasses. It took this hill to prove to me that I need to focus on really seeing things clearly.

Cancer gave me years, more than a decade to identify and pursue my dreams, and time to eradicate my demons. Time—for the first time—to enjoy the wonderful, blessed life I was granted. There are more examples that I could or should state here but here are a few that have stuck with me.

I was given time to see Beth grow and for Greg and Beth to have their first child. The smile on Beth's face when she told us she was expecting is etched in my memory.

Jay, forever imprinted in my mind is the picture of you putting on your national championship hat in Miami; the ear-to-ear smile on your face. That smile gave me thousands of smiles. Oh, how we were both blessed that day.

Daniel, I will always remember two amazing videos. I won't discuss the video of you and James. I still laugh thinking about that mischievous young boy telling the story. The other memory is your presentation on hydrologic fracturing. It was 30± minutes of pure perfection. However, while that was impressive, what I still see, and what was barely visible then, was the clutch cross you were holding. It seemed to give you power. Seeing you that day and on other days when I viewed that video gave me strength.

I now know that I wasn't secure enough in my skin to see what I needed or what I was looking at when I looked at you, Beth, Jay, and Daniel. I know now it was either instantaneous or nearly so that I figured out that you accepted me and understood me.

It was like being struck by lightning. I had learned that my children had accepted me as me. Warts and all. You all gave me the confidence to fight my battle with cancer.

I have a request. It may be hard to fulfill, but please try. Have a party, not a gathering, after the service. Please host the party of a lifetime. Celebrate the life you gave me. Celebrate the joy my family gave me. Know that I'm with mom and dad and my previously departed friends celebrating with you. Let this party be what you remember. Let it be your joy.

Please enjoy every day from here on out, and please smile once a day. Know that my cancer also set you free. I hope I achieved my objective of putting a smile on your face most days. My wish is that you have a smile today, tomorrow, and each day until we see each other again.

Now, please pursue your passion. Know all that I could have ever hoped for was a permanent smile on your face and the faces of our beautiful family.

Know that your dad always loved you and always will.

SURVIVAL JOURNAL ENTRY — OCTOBER 7, 2022

Too Much to Think About

Once again, it's been too long since I have written. There are lots of excuses, but none of them are worthwhile.

It's been a busy time. I had guests most of the year, and for the first time in a long time, I haven't had surgery, unless you call an invasive angiogram surgery. I have two doctors in Jackson that I trust. One was the former head of cardio-oncology at the University of Utah Medical school. She is a major addition to the Jackson medical community.

When I woke up following minor surgery in December 2021, I was told that I had a cardiac event during the procedure. Unlike most people my age, I have a regular workout schedule. I work out six days a week, 30 minutes of Pilates, 30 minutes of light weights, and 30 minutes of aggressive cardio. My resting pulse rate is around 53. When I woke up, I was told about the event and that I had been given too much anesthesia.

I was told that during the procedure, the cardio-oncologist was the M.D. who rescued me. While I was in the hospital, she scheduled follow-up visits. After all, she is a caring, diligent, and highly competent doctor. During each visit, she brought up the need for an angiogram. After several months she convinced me to have the procedure.

Two days after I agreed to the procedure, I was at the University of Utah, where the M.D., who was the most recent head of invasive cardiology at Mass Gen and Harvard Medical School, explained to me about the procedure. I had done my diligence and trusted the doctor. Even after doing that, I was still nervous. Everyone my age seemed to get multiple stents whenever they had an angiogram. I didn't want that because of the restrictions on my activity that would come with blood thinners. I was under the impression that blood thinners may be a lifelong restriction.

When I woke up from the angiogram, the doc told me the procedure was "…much ado about nothing…". He said I had no restriction on blood flow, and to my great relief, he hadn't installed any stints. So, the cardiac event that happened was "much ado about nothing." He also said my heart was good for another 30 years. That comment ended hours of lost sleep and anxiety. However, the anxiety was probably caused and magnified by having two golden retriever puppies.

As some of you know, I have been working on a book about my journey for the past few years. It's been both a labor of love and sometimes a burden. The book's title is "Cancer Set Me Free," and the book is dedicated to:

Those who wish to leave our world and the people, places, and things that occupy it better than we found it.

If I can help others to better weather a journey such as I have, it will be a wonderful endeavor. The good news is that we have a scheduled publication date: Jan 7, 2023. The book will be available on Amazon and at other locations where books are sold.

I have also been working on our book about eclipses. We planned to shoot three eclipses for the book. We shot the Great American Eclipse in 2017 and the Chilean eclipse in 2019. Everything was on track to shoot the Argentina eclipse in 2020, which was on my birthday but then something called covid happened. Well, Argentina wouldn't let us come in, so we looked at shooting the Greenland Eclipse. We were denied entry. So, we settled on shooting the eclipse in Exmouth, Australia, in April 2023. Look it up on a map. 20+ hours of flying followed by a 14-hour car drive. We are dedicated to finishing this book.

If all goes well at the third shoot, we hope to publish our book on eclipses around Oct 1 next year. Please cross your fingers. A 3-year project has turned into a 5-year project. All of you know that one of my many weaknesses is a lack of patience. More truthfully, I am devoid of patience. So here is to a sunny day in Australia.

Before I start this section of the update, I want you to know everything is going to be ok. We all hit potholes, and I am no exception. I appreciate your support and all your offers of assistance. If I need anything, I promise I will ask for it.

I guess I have beaten around the bush long enough. My cancer has not been cooperating. It all started when I had the bright idea that things had been going so well on the 4-week protocol that maybe we should skip a month and find out what would happen. So far, everything that we had done had worked well, so why not try a more reasonable approach?

The "more reasonable approach" didn't go well. The cancer (you may notice I am referring to it as a thinking organism) saw an opening and ran through it with abandon. It started with the development of small tumors and plaques at around the end of the five-week point from my last IV Chemo. My thought was that the new schedule didn't work; let's just go back to the old schedule. Well, that didn't work either. About four weeks ago, it was evident that my cancer was running free. It was like seeing Florida's new quarterback in the secondary with only one slow safety between him and the goal. The moderate approach was no way to materially slow the cancer's growth. So, it was time to amp up the chemo.

I'm now in my 4th month following that dumb mistake, and we have amped up the treatment. Two weeks ago, we more than doubled the daily chemo that I take. This week I had three days of IV Chemo. We also decided that, pending the results of my P.E.T. Scan (which was taken on Tuesday, and we still don't have the results!) that my new schedule is three days of chemo every four weeks. I've also increased the daily chemo again.

If this protocol doesn't work or if the PET provides unwanted results, I will be going to 5 days of IV chemo every three weeks and up to another doubling of my daily chemo.

Again, we are working through a very manageable issue. I was hesitant to write about it, but too many people know what is going on, and I want to prevent well-meaning but inaccurate rumors.

I am ok and will be ok. Remember Sturms Never Quit, That Only You Can Stop You, and We Must All Give Up Hope For a Better Yesterday.

Finally, please do two things for me.

1. Try to put a smile on someone else's face every day; and
2. Please ask yourself, your peers, and coworkers to ask themselves the following question each day on the way home:

What did I do today to make a coworker's job easier or their life better?

Thanks for taking the time to read this post.

Glenn

From my book.

I am now in the second half of my 14th year of chemo. I've had over 500 IV Chemo sessions and over 5,000 days of taking chemo pills. That's just crazy. The only thing I know for sure is that I am blessed. I have been blessed my entire life. I was born in the United States and not in a country like Somalia. I had wonderful grandparents, parents, family, friends, and mentors. I was blessed with a good brain, some artistic talent, and more opportunities than anyone has a right to. I'm blessed to be alive, and I intend to set a record for the most days on chemo in history while Celebrating Life every day. I am truly blessed.

BONUS TIME

I normally get the results from my tests within hours. The longest that I remember it ever took to get results was having to wait until the next day. This time it took a week. As I said earlier, the hardest thing that you have to do is wait. It is one of the things in the process that always creates the highest level of anxiety. And it created a lot of anxiety for me. The longer you wait, the more your mind may start focusing on the worst possible results. Because of the unusual length of time that I had to wait and the recent test results, my anxiety got worse.

I finally got the test results on the patient portal, and I knew enough about my disease to know that they weren't good. Furthermore, when I was able to communicate with my principal oncologist, she said that the PET needed to be reread, so that required more waiting. My next communication was that my doctor needed to talk to an invasive pulmonologist. That wasn't good news.

With that answer, I knew that I had to go to work researching the results of the tests and see what they indicated. Please remember that I'm not a medical doctor and that this is a complicated area. Without going through the machinations of the next week, I sent an article to my Dr. about what I had found, and within 30 minutes, I had a Lung Biopsy scheduled. So, it's another test, and I'm sure another waiting period. I do need to develop more patience.

I don't know the results of the lung biopsy, so my apprehension is probably unwarranted, but I am now getting my chemo for three days every four weeks, and it looks like it may be going to 5 days of infusions every three weeks. As a result of these recent tests and I thought it was a good time to go back and look at the guidance that I have outlined in this book. Sort of doing what I say and doing what I'm doing.

When I wrote "THE CALL," I wrote about an individual who made a lasting impression on me. I said:

I found an article from an individual who died from the disease. He was grateful for the time. He relayed in his article that, unlike his friends who died suddenly in automobile accidents, from heart attacks, or during the war, he had time, and he was grateful for that time. He stated that, while he was dying, he had time to tell his family that he loved them, and he had time to put his issues to rest. While he'd completed his journey some time ago, he taught me that I was just starting my journey, a journey to heal my mind, my body, and my relationships.

I made two statements at the end of my first entry. I said:

You can never imagine how you will react to "the call." I now knew that I was starting a journey, and the destination was mine to decide. While I didn't know how I would conduct myself each day as I faced this journey, I knew that I was creating my destination, and it was going to be great for as long as I had!

I also stated that I wouldn't let cancer define me.

It now looks like I am in bonus time. By all the rules, I should be gone. Heck, I've been in bonus time for almost 15 years. I have so much left to do. I have a 3-year-old grandson who I want to know me. I must shoot the eclipse in Australia next April and then publish my book on eclipses. Heck, I have the Eclipse in Egypt to shoot, and that's in August 2027. That eclipse hits totality at high noon over the Valley of the Kings. I won't miss that. There is so much to do. I know if you pursue a purpose with passion, you will almost always achieve it.

I hope that I have conducted myself in a manner that would make my family proud over the past 14 and ½ years. I will continue to try to improve myself, learn new things, teach others, and make the world a better place than I found it. We can do this by:

- Giving up hope for a better yesterday.
- Never, Never, Ever Quitting
- Putting a smile on someone's face every day.
- Listening, Listening, and Listening before I talk
- Remembering that only you can stop you
- "Knocking it off with them negative waves" (from Kelly's Heroes)
- Remembering that children spell love T.I.M.E
- Remembering that fighting a disease is like climbing a mountain; it can make you stronger if you let it
- Finally, remembering that Cancer Can Set You Free

IN SUMMARY

How do I describe what it's like to grow from having cancer? How do I make having cancer a positive part of my life? I thought of breaking it down into phases. The first phase is generally shock and fear. For me, what followed was (i) rationalization, then (ii) denial, then (iii) education, then (iv) acceptance, then (v) adjustment, and then (vi) lots of other things that include periodical revising of each of the six phases.

You get to a phase when you start looking at the future. During the entire process, you are on a rollercoaster. There are ups and downs. They are not predictable. In some ways, it's like the emotional rollercoaster you were on as a teenager. Sometimes sleep is easy, and sometimes it's impossible. The one thing that I learned was that exercise is the most important part of the treatment. That is until the doctors tell you that you can't exercise at all. So then what do you do? You write about a thirteen plus year battle with cancer and the treatment regimen while summarizing your whole life in a cathartic but monumentally soul-baring expose.

When I go back and read The Call, I realize that I was in shock, denying the disease and its effect on my life and being bewildered by the diagnosis. Why me? What a ridiculous thought. I didn't have anything to do with my cancer unless I made the effect of the cancer worse because of how I reacted to having cancer. I believe that the smartest thing I said in my first posting was:

"You can never imagine how you will react to THE CALL. I now know that I am starting a journey, and the destination is mine to make. While I don't know how I will conduct myself each day as I face this journey, I know that I am creating my destination, and it's going to be a great journey for however long we get."

Each of you and our Divine Creator will be the judge of how I have conducted myself. I believe in forgiveness, and please don't disabuse me of that belief. I know that I have made lots of mistakes, and I regret them all. Even the ones that transported me to a better place. I regret them. They are somewhat like another cancer, but of the spirit. Lingering ghosts that haunt your mind. However, that's the easy part. The hard part is my flaws or the mistakes I don't know about. Things that I have missed that I am blind to or when I don't understand the effect of my actions on others.

Contemplating this writing has caused me once again to think about how I define friends. I believe that to have a friend, you must accept a major flaw in that person. We are all imperfect. We all have flaws, and we may or may not know what they are. Each of you who is reading this will possibly reflect on something that I have done or a tendency that is wrong, even if you don't know me you may be able to read between the lines. You may be focusing on one of my many flaws or, as you now know I like to say, the hole in my swing.

THANK YOU

A s we come to the end of this volume—he says mysteriously while introducing the idea that there could be another book—I would be remiss if I didn't say a special thank you to the special people, the doctors, nurses, and the administrative team at Yale who have supported me over the past ten years. They include:

The professional and administrative staff at Smilow Infusion 7. They include about 40 people. However, two have been there from the first day, and they are Sunshine and Tino (also known as Radar). They are so supportive. Sunshine cares enough to pass the friendship test outlined above. Tino, we missed you more than you could know when you went to Afghanistan as a very young Marine NCO. Semper Fi. If I miss anyone, I apologize; I am doing it all from memory.

Francine Foss, M.D., Professor of Medicine (Hematology) and of Dermatology and until recently Director of Hematology. Thank you for keeping me alive. People ask me why I go to Yale, and I correct them. I go to Dr. Foss. I will go to wherever Dr. Foss is practicing. She is the captain of my ship. She is always thinking. She is always available. One of her most positive skills is that while being completely candid, she is reassuring and develops a protocol that seems individualized. Having absolute confidence in your doctor, specifically your oncologist, in a lot of ways dictates your outcome. I have total and complete confidence in Dr. Foss. I will never be able to thank her enough for my life.

I want to thank Dr. Julie A. Rand-Dorney, M.D. I was referred to her by Richard Kaplan, M.D., during a dark period early in this process. Dr. Rand made a difference for me. Her help and support helped me to develop a positive attitude about cancer. Thank you.

Stacy Hund – 8 years of physical therapy. You have kept me a functional human being. I can still walk without a walker because of your treatment. You are an amazing physical therapist and mom. Congratulations on your new daughter.

Alexandria (Xandi) Garino, PHD, PA-C. You were there on the first day, the day my cancer diagnosis was confirmed. You prepped me for my first meeting with Dr. Foss. You and Dr. Foss confirmed that I had cancer. Your positive attitude and willingness to talk to me at any time gave me the confidence to fight this battle. Thank you. If you can teach a single P.A. to have your people skills each year, you will change the world.

Vikram Reddy, MD, Ph.D., FACS, FASCRS. I don't know what all those initials mean, but your three abdominal surgeries saved my life and gave me a quality of life that I am blessed to have. You have always been available and solved each problem that you presented.

Kevin Becker, M.D., is my neuro-oncologist. Your support and treatment gave me hope. I believe that I can still walk and deal with pain issues without medication because of your help, professional skills, and creativity.

Anna Catino, MD. She saved my life during a surgery during November 2021. Once again I made a mistake, I didn't check out the anesthesiologist. During surgery an issue happened, I had received too much anesthesia. Dr. Catino stepped in and rescued me. She is now a fundamental part of my medical team.

Finally, I want to thank Patty Byrd. She was my executive assistant and colleague for most of my time at my former law firm. She has been a consistent help since I left the firm, sometimes daily. I would be a total mess without her help.

And, of course, my wonderful children. I love you. How lucky I am to have this amazing support system.

My thanks to each and every one of you who has helped me on this journey.

And to the caregivers. All of you. What most people don't understand about cancer is the effect the disease has on the caregiver. I believe that in most cases, the caregivers have a harder time than the patient because everybody worries about the patient, and nobody worries about the caregiver. The caregiver is in a position of absolutely no power, absolutely no authority. It's a selfless job, and it's so hard on them. When you have a friend who has a disease and a caregiver, please help the caregiver. It will make a difference.

In my case, I don't have one of those because I'm single; successfully single, I think. Out of the almost forty five surgeries I've survived, I've only had people physically present at two of them, which is kind of unusual. Sometimes its been easier for me to do it alone.

It would be antithetical to write the words "The End" here, so I'll just simply say, "That's all for now," thanks for reading.

Glenn

Follow Glenn's journey as it continues on www.GlennSturm.com

Printed in the USA
CPSIA information can be obtained
at www.ICGtesting.com
CBHW031052261123
1820CB00037B/38/J